Praise for Parenting Our Parents

"A must-read for children of aging parents. Jane Wolf Frances writes from a firm base of empathy and knowledge about a situation that—sooner or later—affects us all. Her book provided me with trustworthy companionship and practical guidance in just the right amounts. Extremely useful and highly recommended." **—Darcie Sanders**, trustee, Lyons Regional Library District; co-author of *Staying Home*

"A brilliant, heartfelt, and very personal book that I believe will become indispensable to a great many people. It is filled with important information from a woman who has gained this wisdom the hard way. If you are in this parenting role or about to be, this is the place to start." **—Rick Moss**, PhD, minister of religious science; developer of Awakening to Our Greatness

"As a caregiver for ten years and a gerontologist, I wish I had had this book at the beginning of my journey. Reading this was highly comforting and made me consider the honor it gives me to take care of my father. I feel blessed that I have the opportunity to savor it." **—Maria Siciliano**, MSG, MPA, principal and founder of Gerontology in Action

"*Parenting Our Parents* takes the guesswork out of parenting older relatives and loved ones by helping the reader make informed decisions and offering both tools for communication and plans for going forward at a time when confusion and denial can run rampant. Her 'how-to' guide offers a process and understanding that can make this daunting journey not just bearable but truly an act of love. " **—Patricia Mitchell**, broadcaster, life coach, and consultant, Certified POP Family Coach

"This book is a revelation, a generous, comprehensive, and wise guided tour of all the issues we confront in struggling to meet the needs of aging and increasingly dependent parents. It's loaded with wisdom, practical advice, and inspiration on everything I and my family faced as our parents aged, got sick, and faced death, needing their kids more and more." —**Holly Knox**, instructional designer (retired)

"Frances has written an extraordinarily valuable book for so many people who currently or will eventually care for their parents. She is an empathetic instructor who can help others with the difficulties of recognizing the signs that our parents need help and following through with those decisions that affect the lives of both parties. People *need* to read this book and keep it close—it will aid their hearts and minds and enrich their lives." —**Rikki Klieman**, attorney and legal analyst

PARENTING OUR PARENTS

PARENTING OUR PARENTS

Transforming the Challenge into a Journey of Love

Jane Wolf Frances, JD, MSW

ROWMAN & LITTLEFIELD
Lanham • Boulder • New York • London

Published by Rowman & Littlefield
An imprint of The Rowman & Littlefield Publishing Group, Inc.
4501 Forbes Boulevard, Suite 200, Lanham, Maryland 20706
www.rowman.com

6 Tinworth Street, London SE11 5AL, United Kingdom

British Library Cataloguing in Publication Information Available

Library of Congress Cataloging-in-Publication Data Is Available

ISBN 978-1-5381-2796-4 (cloth: alk. paper)
ISBN 978-1-5381-2797-1 (electronic)

♾ ™ The paper used in this publication meets the minimum requirements of American National Standard for Information Sciences Permanence of Paper for Printed Library Materials, ANSI/NISO Z39.48-1992.

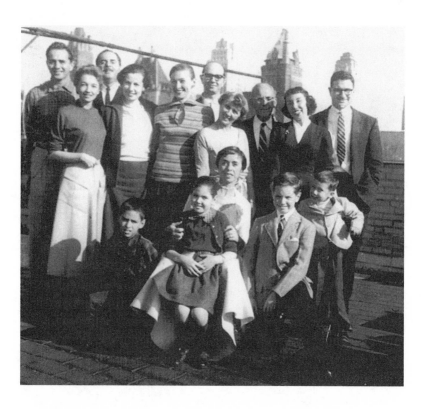

Family photo of Dad's four living Wolf siblings and families, including my childhood close cousins: Rick, to my right, later to become my "adopted brother"; Dick, to my left, later to create *Law & Order*.

CONTENTS

PROLOGUE

Why I Wrote This Book

That Christmas vacation, when I first caught sight of my folks and saw how much they had aged, and then saw the dirt and disorder that had taken over their formerly immaculate home, I knew two things. The first was that my parents needed assistance. But almost as clearly, I saw that I, too, would need help, and lots of it.

Although I had no idea then how much help I'd need or where that help would come from, I did sense that something very different was happening and that major changes were ahead. As events unfolded, that prediction proved alarmingly accurate. It was a life-changing moment, and neither I nor Mom and Dad would ever be quite the same again.

My parents, Lillian and Jack Wolf, were then eighty-five years old and living as they always had—in their home, "independently." But I was no longer their teenage daughter doing my homework down the hall. I'd grown up and moved a continent away many years before. Recently, in midlife, I'd returned to graduate school in order to begin a second career. Earlier that winter, I was very busy building my new practice as a psychotherapist, working with seniors and their families. I'd been excited to share all about that with my parents.

You might imagine that someone with my background would have been better at predicting that my parents and I would have "some accommodating" to do as we all aged. Somehow, I'd managed to plan ahead for very little of that and instead lived with, in hindsight, a surprising level of denial. The bald truth was that I was an only child and my folks were octogenarians who lived thousands of miles away from me. What could possibly go wrong?

Although it seems unimaginable that my parents would conceal their health or other problems from me, it's not at all uncommon for older parents to do so. Like Jack and Lillian, many of your parents might have fears of the unknown consequences of "inviting" their family in to help them and, instead, resort to hiding things from you. Once I saw for myself what was really happening with my folks, I had to play catch-up, not having planned as well as I could have nor dealt with my nagging concerns for their health.

When I got past my initial reaction I was able to take a breath. By doing that, I found I could respond rather than react: one of the first tools of good parenting, as it turns out. Then I was able to look more deeply. I discovered that my parents' needs were vast and pressing. It became apparent that I would need to not only make sense of what was happening medically but also step in to deal with a whole laundry list of nonmedical issues for them. Before long, I was wishing I could have taken care of things earlier, but I at least recognized that I now had to try to solve problems that, even a day before, I hadn't considered to be mine.

When I found a few moments to come up for air, I instinctively turned to books and the internet, my usual sources for comprehensive information and perspective. I was searching for an "expert" to tell me how to become a more caring and involved daughter at this time of my parents' life. As a specialist myself in the field of geriatric psychotherapy, I was familiar with the literature on aging, death, and loss. I'd always regretted that there wasn't a really good book—not even a helpful magazine article on "raising" older parents, nothing useful on television or the web—to recommend to my patients as they traversed the journey my parents and I now apparently had begun. In the past, I'd wanted to offer "biblio-therapy"[1]—intelligent, empathic literature—to further help my patients steer their courses during this part of life.

Now it was I who was feeling confused, lonely, and bereft: I needed guidance of my own!

I was beginning to understand that I would need to take on a different role with Jack and Lillian, one requiring the skills and qualities I generally associated with good parenting. I was desperately seeking some smart professor's book or reputable organization's research study to help me make sense of what this new role and my new job would entail. But nothing was out there. I considered that perhaps this new relationship with my parents was, in fact, all about parenting. This was a new type of parenting, however, parenting that appeared in a radically different context. It was "parenting" by adult children who had "turned it around" by deciding to care for elderly parents who, so long ago, had cared for them.

I could even see ahead to the day when this role reversal would be fully realized: many of us would quite naturally be "Parenting Our Parents" (or "doing POP," for short). It was then that I first came to realize for the first time that the book I was so longing for was one I might actually need to write. I would write it to guide me and you and hopefully to mentor generations through the phase of a hitherto-unnamed twenty-first-century developmental stage of life I called the POPcycle.

The term "POPcycle" describes with eerie precision what happened over time in my family and what occurs in most other families. The POPcycle starts when the older generation begins to cede some decision-making and control to those in the younger generation, the adult children who simultaneously find themselves taking on more and more responsibility for many aspects of their aging parents' (and other beloved relatives') lives.

Dr. Benjamin Spock's *Baby and Child Care*[2] famously comforted generations of young parents, starting with my own, by educating them to the predictable stages of their children's developmental cycle. Similarly, the popular *What to Expect When*

You're Expecting[3] was heralded by decades of soon-to-be parents for guiding them through the developmental stages of pregnancy.

I saw that what people parenting their parents needed was such a book for our generation's new "assignment." What I'd tried so hard to find unsuccessfully was a handbook to guide me through the hardest parenting challenge of all: "POParenting" or parenting those people who'd raised me. I would have been over-joyed to have even found a magazine about parenting our parents, like the dozens I'd seen for parenting our kids. I still vividly recall my aloneness and yearning for connection, community, and a book that would include but also go beyond a simple "how-to" book approach. My patients and I needed something to guide us be-yond the activities of basic caregiving, picking up prescriptions, and creating viable health care proxies. We needed a book that would help us find the meaning, healing, and joy of doing POP.

What I saw I also needed was a book that would address the overwhelming emotions both sides of those in the POPcycle so often reported feeling. For the middle-agers, there is an incred-ible sense of aloneness, as if we were the only ones doing POP; there are fears associated with not doing it right and often there are old or current family resentments that make POParenting par-ticularly challenging. And for the senior parents, there is a fear of losing our independence and "voice," of the loneliness associated with the death of mates and friends, and often the emotional and physical readjustments that accompany "leaving home."

Some of my patients who were the most interested in a com-prehensive book were elder patients themselves. Appreciating that their bodies and minds and their relationships with their adult children were changing, savvy seniors wanted to educate them-selves—as well as their children—about how to best navigate the POPcycle they would be sharing. They wanted four books, one for themselves and three more for their grown offspring, they'd tell me.

Still hoping I could find someone else's book, I aimed to find a memoir that might illustrate a micro-view, something up close and personal I could learn from. I'd thought that maybe by reading another person's story, I could more easily create the vision of how to do POP in my own family. At other times, I'd wanted to locate a treatise on "How to Care for Your Mom and Dad While Still Having Your Own Life" to better balance my new POP responsibilities on top of everything else already on my plate. How was this going to work: adding Jack and Lillian's concerns to my existing stressors, to everyone else competing for my time and attention? I'd also wanted to find something with a macro-view, as if I were standing up high on a movie director's crane. From there, maybe I could better "oversee" POP for the phenomenon it had become, something being replicated in millions of homes across this nation and beyond, but especially in the United States with our seemingly shrinking "safety net" beneath America's aging families.

I wondered: If I, with my years of geriatric training and experience, was feeling so lonely and "clueless," how would someone without all my background and expertise cope?

Eventually, I knew that the only way to have such a resource for others was to sit down and write the book I'd so desperately wanted but never been able to find. My intention in doing so was to make your Parenting Our Parents (POP) experience and that of many others easier, more comprehensible and, yes, more enjoyable than mine had been for me.

Since that attention-grabbing Christmas in 1997, when my family's POPcycle began, of course an awful lot has occurred. You and I now have the internet and the electronic world, replacing books for many as their primary source of information. The web's capability to instantaneously and continuously connect us to each other as well as vast quantities of information has created extraordinary opportunities, ones with potential to bring together and invigorate communities online. Hmmm . . . my wheels continued to turn.

While working on this book, my concern for the fragmented and fragile social net under our nation's most susceptible demographic, our seniors, continued to grow. I began to see an expanded vision, one far bigger than any single family's journey. I came to realize that those of us doing POP needed even more than a really good book. What we also required, it seemed, was a POP community, a movement that would provide momentum, energy, and involvement. The support of others could successfully equip us to fulfill the enormous responsibilities and accomplish the tasks of POP, of parenting our own parents.

I began to imagine: What if those who choose to complete the Circle of Life by Parenting Our Parents, create our own POP community? A POP community would help us "support ourselves" and our fellow POParents as well. It could offer us information, advice, inspiration, and online invitations to events. It could show us how to "do POP" by giving us examples, provide us models of good (or not-so-good) POParenting to learn from. Maybe the government wouldn't need to set up new institutions or provide additional benefits if we created a POP community that worked well enough to yield our own safety net? I'd have been ecstatic to have discovered a way to "chat" online with others who, like me, who were wide awake at 3 a.m. trying to figure out how to install grab bars before our parents returned from their postsurgical rehabilitation the next day.

When you're next awake at 3 a.m. worrying about your parents and how you'll best cope, no one from the government will be by your side helping to solve your latest POP problem. Now, however, you'll possess two other very useful things close by. You will have your copy of this book, *Parenting Our Parents: Transforming This Challenge into a Journey of Love* and you'll have your own friends and POP community at www.ParentingOurParents.org.

The website is based on the premise that all of us doing POP have much to teach and much to learn from each other, and we all do some of each—teaching and learning—in the POP community. At the website, you'll have access to extraordinary POParents 24/7. POParents are people from families like yours, working to make this a time of safety, healing, order, and joy for everyone involved. The POP community consists of geriatric "experts" and compassionate POParents, people like you and me, interested in healing the wounds of our past and creating loving family experiences in our present and for our future.

Writing this book presented "impediments" that were unknown to me when I began, much like parenting my parents had done. One of my biggest challenges was publicly sharing the intimacies of my family's POP journey. My folks had always guarded their privacy zealously, like so many of their generation. And even though my parents passed before this book was published, I sometimes felt that telling "My Story" revealed too much of our family's "secrets." Eventually, I came to realize that my parents would have been proud of me, as they always were, for using our family's experiences to help others.

Another challenge is that customarily in the practice of my psychotherapy profession, it's the patient revealing his or her life story, not the therapist revealing hers. I had to come to accept that I needed to step outside that comfortable "anonymous zone" and allow you to authentically know me and my family: by doing so, my words would gain real credibility in your eyes and therefore be of most help.

So why did I write this book and start this POP community? I did so because I wanted to support you and others like you in manifesting your vision of POP love and loyalty. By being part of this new POP community, we are positively altering the face and character of our nation in how we treat our aging population. Should this book and the POP community help you transform your family relationships into ones you've always wanted, you and I will have made a significant contribution to there being more joy in your life and the lives of your loved ones and our nation.

I

FINDING OUT OUR PARENTS NEED SOMEONE TO HELP THEM

MY STORY

During the previous few years, it hadn't simply been my desire to spend time with my parents that led me to make more trips cross-country. Instead, a protracted illness plaguing Mom for "just too long" or an unexpected angiogram that Dad needed were the specific factors that motivated me to leave home in Southern California for New York City, especially during the bracing winter months. Even then, my visits to see Mom and Dad were neither as habitual nor as frequent as they would soon become.

When I came to town that life-changing December, it had only been a matter of months since I'd seen them last. Ever since I'd left home for college, my parents had always been so excited to see their only child that they would come and pick me up from whatever airport I flew into rather than wait for a taxi to deliver me to their apartment. But this visit, in the freezing night air, no one was at the airport for me.

Not only was there no warm welcome, but when I called them on the phone from the hotel where soon I would become a regular, Dad was curt, monosyllabic, and distant. That was so unlike him. Also, sounding extraordinarily exhausted, he tried putting off getting together for dinner until the last possible moment. It seemed as if Dad wished I would cancel the evening entirely.

When I finally met up with Lillian and Jack Wolf at a cozy neighborhood restaurant that unnerving evening, I didn't recognize the old, worn-down couple in front of me. Having always known her to be a perfectionist, Mom's appearance was shocking. She looked like someone had pulled some old dress from the back of her closet and stuffed her into it. Mom's customary hairstyle—immaculately combed and carefully organized into a white-haired bun—appeared to have had a comb half-heartedly dragged through it. My hitherto elegant mother would never have let herself out of the house looking like that.

In other ways too, she was a shadow of her former self. Mom's breathing was clearly labored as she dragged herself to our table at a glacial pace. When I kissed her cheek, her skin was eerily cold to the touch. My sense was that she was icy from the inside all the way to the surface, not merely chilled by the cold temperatures outside.

Earlier in the week, when we'd spoken on the phone, I detected nothing unusual, but the woman in front of me could hardly formulate whole sentences. She had difficulty following our conversation and couldn't focus on the ordinary restaurant tasks of reading a menu and ordering. When she allowed Dad to order her meal and then speak for her, I knew something was seriously amiss. My "real" mother would never have heard of such a thing.

Dad was acting nothing like his normal self either. He radiated fatigue of such a deep nature that no amount of sleep looked like it would restore him. When I was still back in L.A. talking to him long distance, his voice had been able to deceive me. He had successfully concealed this complete exhaustion—physical, emotional, and mental—but now in person, I could see the true nature of his condition. One of Dad's signature characteristics was his fascination with life's details and his daughter; in my dating years, often I'd had to pry my boyfriends away from talking to him. But that night, Jack showed little interest in anything.

As I lay tossing and turning in bed later that night, I couldn't deny that there was something very troubling going on. I'd wanted to chalk up my parents' disturbing ways to "a bad evening." Certainly, we all have them, I told myself. But I just kept thinking: Who stole my parents? Who were these doddering people?

I tried playing detective by thinking back to their histories. Generally, Mom had been as healthy and energetic as women years younger. However, a few years before, she'd contracted a case of pneumonia serious enough to require hospitalization. During that stay, some attending doctor while conducting rounds informed me by long-distance telephone that Mom had dementia of the Alzheimer's type. It was a diagnosis I'd questioned at the time due to the tests he'd used and other factors, like her being disoriented in an unfamiliar hospital setting. But lying in bed, I wondered if what I was seeing now could be Alzheimer's?

In 1974 I moved to California from the East Coast, where I'd been raised and schooled. By the time I made this holiday visit in 1997, I'd lived out West for nearly twenty-five years. I was approaching middle age and my parents were each eighty-five. Although I'd seen aspects of Mom's memory dimming during earlier visits, I was shocked when that doctor broke the news to me of his medical opinion. Watching her work her beloved crossword puzzles for many years following this diagnosis supported my suspicion that it had never been properly determined.

However, on this sleepless night of searching for a reasonable explanation of her bizarre behavior, I feared that Mom was finally "showing her Alzheimer's." Understanding the slow and progressive course of the disease as I did from years of working as a geriatric therapist, I soon ruled out that dementia had suddenly descended on my poor mother. It wasn't possible that she had declined so rapidly as to need institutionalization, between the time on Monday when she'd talked lucidly on the telephone and Friday when I saw her in the restaurant. There must be something else going on. As for Dad, I thought that perhaps he too had gotten sick while caring for and worrying about Mom. I was troubled by his appearance and lack of spirit as well.

My most pressing problem was to discover what was causing them to seem so unlike themselves—so very old and needy. The next morning, bleary-eyed from lack of sleep, I called to arrange to have breakfast with them. Dad put me off, postponing our getting together that day completely. "Mom's still under the weather," he said casually. "Go enjoy your friends and the wonderful show at the Met." The following morning, I called again and got more excuses. In fact, Dad seemed more determined than ever that I stay away.

A part of me wanted to obey him and let them rest alone. But another part just couldn't do the "good daughter" thing and comply, because something wasn't right. Once I'd made up my mind that I needed to see for myself what was going on, the taxi-ride across town seemed to take forever. The look on my father's face when he opened the door to their apartment, and his cold stare were both foreign to me: "I told you not to come. What are you doing here?" Once inside, the sight left me in shock, stone cold. It wasn't long before sad and even mad joined the emotion of shock.

My mother, always so attentive to the appearance of her home, herself and her things, had allowed their apartment to become caked with dust. I quickly calculated that that much dust must have taken a while to accumulate. I learned as I walked in that my folks had gotten rid of their longtime housekeeper at a time when they particularly needed someone to clean and cook for them. Nostalgically, I remembered how Dad used to joke that Mom was so neat "she'd make the bed in the middle of the night, even before I returned from the bathroom." That seemed like a lifetime ago.

Heading into their bedroom, I saw that my venerable parents were sleeping in sheets that had turned a deep gray from their original white. Neither of them had taken a bath in several weeks, as it turned out. Mom had been too weak to navigate the tub and Dad was afraid to leave her alone long enough to bathe himself. Predictably, their moods were equally low. Mom was confused, alternately passive and then aggressive, even lashing out violently if she felt she was being challenged.

Dad seemed deeply disturbed, not only by his own fatigue, but perhaps more pressingly by his inability to care for his sick wife and whatever meaning he was attaching to that. It all seemed to be dangerously depressing him. I finally understood why my father hadn't wanted me to come over. They both had been hiding from me the extent of their medical conditions, their home, and their need for help! In that moment, I feared for all of us, for myself as well as for them. Things had gotten totally out of control and someone needed to straighten them out.

There was no one but me. I had no siblings or even close friends who lived near enough to enlist for the type of help I was now envisioning my parents were going to need. I previously had no plans to stop working; quite the opposite, as I had just started my second career thousands of miles away. Although surrounded by my clearly dependent parents, I suddenly felt alone. And in spite of my years of seemingly relevant education and experience, I was lost and panicky.

I saw that I'd been pretty much ignoring the fact that someday my parents would need help. I had been reluctant to ask them important questions until this crisis forced me to. Up until that visit, I had avoided looking ahead and had made no plans for my parents' future. Now I needed to do a lot of fast thinking and catching up. My New York vacation had been scheduled to end in three more days, when I was slated to return to my life in California.

What life? My life—as I'd known it up until then—seemed like it was about to be altered forever. Slowly I saw there were significant choices I would need to make. Would my attention, time, and resources become increasingly trained on my parents? It seemed I might be choosing to honor and preserve the threesome my life had begun with or that "'til death do us part" might refer to my new relationship with my parents. I might even have to contemplate parenting my own parents as my commitment grew over time.

Was I ready and willing to parent my own parents? They seemed to need something different from me than I'd ever considered before. If I decided to care for Lillian and Jack, I might have to give up many of my previous pictures of how my life was supposed to be. I would need to make important decisions, maybe different ones than I'd previously expected.

I didn't yet know that I would find myself maneuvering through complicated role reversals, balancing my need for my parents' safety with their independence, and discovering how to honor both their wishes as well as my own. I couldn't even imagine how long caring for my parents might last or what kinds of changes I would need to face. Nor did I realize at that moment that I'd remain on call and never leave a phone unanswered for the next ten years lest I miss an urgent call from my parents or their doctors.

But I'm getting ahead of myself. On that freezing December morning that marked the birth of our family's POPcycle, there were no tree ornaments or other symbols to suggest any festivities at the Wolf home. Instead, that morning initiated an intense nos-

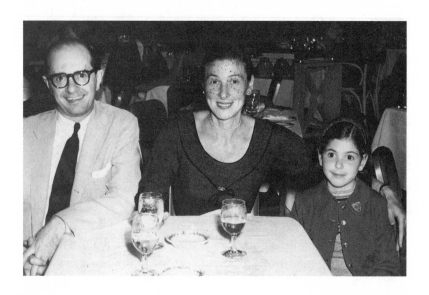

Figure 1.1.   Young Jane at five out celebrating a birthday with my Mommy and Daddy

talgia, as the girl in me longed for the old days, when things were fine. It felt like I was going through the rigors of birthing a new phase of my life. Maybe more importantly, in that moment, it felt like death—the end of an era.

If I were to take on this challenge, Lillian, Jack, and I would need to reverse our roles. I would be caring for them this time around. That Christmas, we were beginning our last journey together, through a cycle that would be unidirectional and irreversible. I could see ahead enough to imagine the way it would go: my parents would inevitably become increasingly unable to care for themselves and the details of their lives. They would become more and more dependent on me. Simultaneously, I would become more and more responsible for them, making more and more of their decisions and acting increasingly parental.

THEIR STORY—DAD

Since Lillian had started coughing and wheezing, maybe two weeks earlier, she had become weaker and was acting more bizarrely each day. I too had come down with something physically unpleasant, a tickle in my throat and some sneezing, but I avoided taking my temperature. Instead, I just kept popping aspirin. I saw it as my responsibility to look after Lillian, after all I always had.

When we'd first met, taking care of Lillian had been all I'd wanted. Our fit seemed a natural. Not only was she a strikingly beautiful and smart woman, she was also the youngest in a family of six, vulnerable from having lost her dad as a mere girl of five. I was the eldest son and I had always protected my younger brothers—organizing the boys, making sure everyone had enough food and pocket money and that their homework was done. My father didn't pay that much attention to us kids. That was the way at the time. My mother was absent a lot, having been a political activist and a newspaper columnist. So, I learned to do a lot of family caregiving from the time I was fairly young. Probably it was also in my nature.

I had thought that looking after Lillian now, with her coughing and weakness, would be fairly simple. I'd bring her what she needed—some aspirin, something to help her breathe better, some chicken soup—but nothing I did was helping her much. My wife seemed to be getting worse rather than better. I didn't really know what to do.

As Lillian's physical condition worsened, her behavior also became increasingly irrational. She had been insistent that I not tell Jane how ill she had become. When I suggested we invite Jane over to help us since she was in town, Lillian's response had been immediate: "Absolutely not! She'll just want to come in here and tell me what to do," Lillian had cried. I didn't know what to do but decided to keep my wife calm by agreeing with her. Usually that worked.

The night we met Jane for dinner at the restaurant was our first venture out of our apartment in some weeks. It took a lot out of both of us. For days we hadn't really bathed or changed our clothes very often. I didn't have enough strength to lift Lillian high enough to get her into or out of our bathtub although we both did need to wash, after a while. When I reached the point where I knew I needed to bathe, I was afraid to leave her alone long enough to run my own tub and soak there. So, I just kept waiting, thinking eventually it would all pass and things would return to normal. I was so exhausted I often couldn't sleep. My body and mind were beyond any fatigue I'd ever known, or at least as I can recall at this point.

In order to go out to meet Jane for dinner, I'd been forced to get some clean clothes on Lillian and myself and to straighten her hair out as well. She would barely let me put a comb through her beautiful white hair, generally perfectly organized, but that night it looked all ratted up and silly. I have hardly any hair of my own, so tending hers was not something I did well. Dressing her was another matter. I found a dress in her closet that she used to like wearing, but she wasn't very cooperative. When I was done, she looked amazingly disheveled, as if someone had poured her into someone else's dress. I thought to change her but didn't have the energy to start all over again.

I know Jane was taken aback that first night when she saw us both, especially Lillian. My approach was just to get us through the evening—order for Lillian, eat, and make some conversation. I was so stressed just trying to make everything seem normal. I was still hoping that pacifying Lillian would get us beyond this particular crisis and then we'd be able to get back home without Jane's becoming too suspicious.

Putting Jane off for a day or two after that dinner seemed to work. But then she showed up unexpectedly at our front door, after I'd told her specifically not to come. Finding Jane there was a shock. Her mother and I had always encouraged her to have a mind of her own and I'd been proud to see her develop as a bright and independent thinker. But Jane was also an obedient girl, having given us no real trouble and doing what we'd asked of her most of the time, as far as I knew. That morning was the first time I remember her ever defying me directly. While we were on the phone I'd said clearly to my daughter: "Do not come here," but hardly were the words even out of my mouth, she was at our door.

I wouldn't have tried to keep the state of Lillian's ill health or our home from Jane if it had been totally up to me. I thought Lillian's dissembling was ill conceived, especially since Jane was coming to town and, most certainly, would observe the condition of our apartment and our health. But Lillian had always been concerned to be her own person and had some fear that Jane would take that away: she had also become increasingly paranoid as her illness wore on. I had been torn, wanting Jane to know but not wanting to upset Lillian.

And then all of a sudden, Jane was there at our door. I felt like we'd been caught red-handed. After my shock and short-lived anger retreated, I recognized that I was enormously relieved I didn't have to hide anything anymore. The truth Jane saw was not pretty. Lillian had always been a perfectionist about her home and her appearance and a really clean person. But she had begun to let everything go. She didn't open the mail or clean a dish. Things were just used and then left everywhere. The dust was caked on our beautiful antiques she and I had so carefully chosen years before. I understood how badly my wife must have been feeling to let everything go like this. To Jane, the current scene was the exact opposite of her childhood home: it must have been frightening.

We hadn't changed the sheets or done laundry in a while either, so Lillian and I were sleeping on pretty badly graying sheets. Everything was becoming harder and harder to take care of. Things were piling up around us. I had taken to calling in for our meals from our favorite delis and coffee shops in the neighborhood, so we did stay fed. As for me, I was desperate to see Lillian's special smile reappear and I would have done anything to bring it back.

Now that Jane had seen fit to defy me and show up, I knew that she would help me.

YOUR STORY

If you are fortunate enough to still have older living parents or other close loved ones who are seniors, you must have seen them change over time. Whether your attention was drawn to this slowly and imperceptibly through the years or dramatically one day, you must have seen that, after a while, even the most robust of our elders starts to slow down.

Not everyone has as dramatic or traumatic a Christmas "revelation story" as I did, thankfully. Maybe you first noticed the change when your parents uncharacteristically began asking you for advice—and then actually took it. Or maybe your folks simply started expecting you to help them with many more things, far more often than they used to. Perhaps it was your mother-in-law's continued refusal to accept your help when she clearly needed it that caught your eye.

Maybe your mom took a fall a few months ago and even though she's tried, she can't really get back on her feet. Now maybe she's having trouble going back to work and even getting to the market.

Cooking, which she'd always loved, is becoming a chore. She's feeling badly that she can't take care of your kids on Saturdays, as she used to. According to the Centers for Disease Control and Prevention, three million older Americans are treated in ERs from fall injuries. The long-term impact of such falls can often be life changing for the senior and the family (see https://www.cdc.gov/homeandrecreationalsafety/falls/adultfalls.html).

Or perhaps your wake-up call came in the form of your dad's calling you, incensed about some man repeatedly phoning him about some unpaid hospital bill who is getting increasingly hostile. Although he doesn't remember being hospitalized, your dad would like this bill paid just to stop the disturbing phone calls. Maybe he did pay the bill, he tells you. He's not really sure if he's been in a hospital recently or not, so he asks you to speak to the man for him.

Maybe your parents have recently stopped coming to Sunday-night dinners at your house. At first, they offered weak excuses, but one day your mom finally revealed: "Dad doesn't like to drive at night anymore." On a hunch, on your next visit to your parents' home, you take a look at his vintage car and notice the passenger door is dented and the car has a flat tire. You understand that it's more than night driving your father is no longer doing. You wonder if he's been afraid to drive or if he even should. Did he have an accident? Was anyone hurt? Is there a lawsuit pending? Is he confused on the road? Is he afraid to tell you that he dented the car? Maybe he really wants you to know. You ask a few more questions and find out: "I had a small accident. I didn't think you needed to know."

These are the sort of telltale signs that can let you know that your parents are beginning to need some help. The people who raised you may now need you and/or your siblings or even an occasional caregiver to do a few tasks so everything can "get back to normal." But your parents, like mine, will continue to slow down and progressively age. And eventually, if they live long enough, your parents may resemble childlike, even infantile, versions of their earlier selves. You are witnessing the final chapter in their life, the POPcycle.

As you pay further attention to these initial signs of aging and stop to evaluate your parents' level of frailty, fragility, or even possible senility, you may also be catching a glimpse of a unique part of your own life cycle. If you also choose to parent your own parents, you will be joining a special cadre of loving people who are taking on more and more responsibility for their aging parents' well-being.

Soon you may be taking your parents to their doctor appointments, where you may often act as their historians, truth tellers, and translators. Then you will probably find yourself interceding for your parents with Medicare and Social Security. Next, you're getting their perhaps all-too-numerous prescriptions filled and refilled and picking up some adult diapers—since you're already at the pharmacist. And before long, you're paying their delinquent, "misplaced" bills and shopping for healthier food for them. And one bizarre day, soon, you may be telling the very people from whom you used to borrow the family car that they need to stop driving.

Many of you have already begun attending to your aging parents, some full-time and some part-time. Your involvement is at some point likely to become critical to your parents' everyday living. The truth is that you and I are developing new relationships with our senior parents, ones we probably never expected we would have. Over the course of time, you are likely to become substantially involved in your parents' lives emotionally, financially, and even spiritually. Some of you may leave your job, give up your home, and move across states to POParent your folks. Given the longevity of today's seniors and the current offering of new medical treatments and pharmaceuticals, no matter how many years you put in to parent your children, you may end up parenting your parents for even longer.

If you choose to parent your parents, you will be joining me and countless others who've made the choice—to Parent Our Parents, to do POP. You will be part of the millions of loving adult children who are deciding that we wish to devote ourselves to caring for our aging relatives and making this POP time a special one for all concerned. Your realization of your parents' neediness and your need to face this decision may be as shocking as mine was. Ultimately, you may join us in saying: *Oh my God! We're Parenting Our Parents! We're doing POP!*

Choosing to do POP at this important juncture can provide unexpected opportunities for completion and closure for you, your other family members, and certainly for your parents. How you choose to participate in this special time is limited only by your particular circumstances and your imagination. Some will make up for missed time from the past. Others will establish more intimate connections with their parents than they've ever had before. Still others will undo decades-long estrangements with their parents and siblings.

How will you know if your time for doing POP has begun? How might your parents display their changes to you? How can you learn to read the signs soon enough so that, hopefully, you will have figured this out before you face the kind of crisis I encountered? Will you be able to demonstrate the necessary confidence, courage, and determination to discover whether, how much, and when your parents need POParenting?

You will need a method to evaluate your parents' needs, both at the start and then again later. Likely you will have to do so repeatedly over your years of doing POP. To help you better conceptualize what is happening developmentally between you and your parents, their growing dependency, and your increased responsibility and decision-making, I offer you the "POPcycle" (not necessarily pronounced "Popsicle").

You can chart the relevant factors in your senior parents' functional dependence/independence to see when, where, and how you will want or need to increase the support and protection for your aging loved ones. It is useful to have the POPcycle as a measurement of where your parents are, since the chronological model that pediatricians use to assess your child's development is of little value to the geriatrician or the POP family seeking to evaluate aging parents' development.

Once you've done your initial assessment of your parents' current circumstances, you will need to discover many other important things. You will either choose to jump in or else find out if there is or could be someone else to take on the job. But for that, you will want to move on to chapter 2.

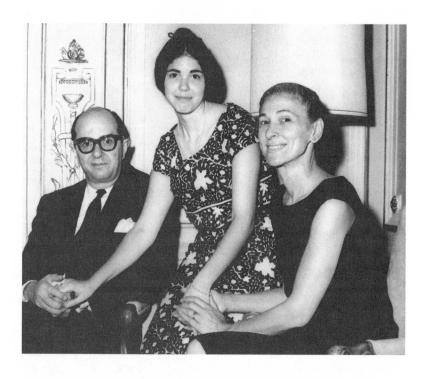

Figure 1.2. Sweet sixteen with my fifty-ish-year-old parents

2

CHOOSING POP—OR NOT

MY STORY

After accepting the irrefutable fact that my parents needed serious help and that it should have started yesterday, I attempted to process the additional fact that they'd been actively concealing the state of their affairs from me. Me, of all people! I found myself flooded with all sorts of feelings, memories, thoughts, and questions. I decided to let my mental meanderings lead me wherever they took me. But I knew enough not to necessarily use them as the basis for my decision of whether I'd choose to do POP.

When I was seventeen years old I moved out of my parents' apartment in New York City and went off to dorm life at Wellesley College. It was located in the suburbs of Boston, about a four-hour drive from my parents' home. In high school they'd warned us that we would be little fish in a big pond at college. So, when I got there, I studied long, hard, and often. I became a history major because I was fascinated to understand how people managed their lives at other times and in other places. I also widened my window on the world by living on my own, away from my folks and their daily influence. At Wellesley, I was surrounded by the new friends I met there, women with whom I was beginning lifelong relationships, people who would impact me more than the studies I'd come there for—people I still cherish and rely on for their advice and love, long after my parents have gone.

Following my undergraduate years, I spent three more years continuing my education at the Boston University School of Law. There I specialized in the emerging field of poverty law, since I wished to be a part of making our world and our country a fairer place to live. My becoming a lawyer and fighting for the rights of the poor gave me a bird's-eye view on how tough life can be for the underdog in the United States. Later in life, when I focused my concerns on what was happening with the elderly, I came to see the parallel: our older parents, especially those with disabilities and chronic illness had, in many ways, joined the ranks of the underdogs in our country.

During the 1960s and 1970s, when many baby boomers were completing schooling and starting careers, California was regarded as a Mecca. It represented the cutting edge of what was evolving in our country—politically, musically, culturally, and socially.

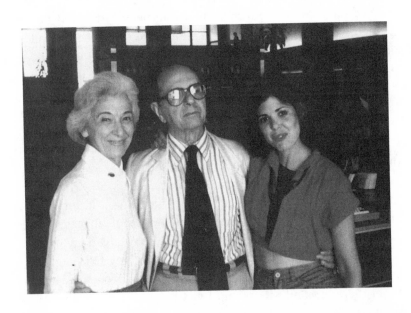

Figure 2.1.   Mom and Dad in their early seventies visiting me in California

Some were lured out to California by the promise of a climatic paradise, others by the freethinking and free living; many went for careers. I'd long dreamed of living in the sunny and inviting state, even of driving a convertible where I could rock and bop to the radio on the highways they called freeways.

When the pull of work led me to California, I made those dreams into my reality. After three years of practicing law in Boston, I joined those who were placing even larger distances between themselves and their parents, moving all the way to the West Coast. Beyond the attraction of the geography, many were also expressing an alienation that stemmed from a clash with our parents' generation over a variety of choices they'd made. My generation held on to both a sense of hope—that we could create a different world, a better world than those who'd tried before us—and a sense of despair, having seen our leaders assassinated and our peers killed in a war we watched on TV during dinner.

My parents' cultural values—love and marriage and being able to rely on a caring family—was something they held in common with each other and shared with me. I don't imagine any of us expected those principles to play out or affect us in the way they did, so many years after I left their home.

It was largely because of those values, because of who my parents were and how they'd raised me, that I was now choosing to parent them, the ones who'd parented me. It would not be a smooth road for any of us, as you will soon read, but the worth of our life experiences isn't necessarily a function of its ease.

My parents met back in 1940 when my mother brought a dirty dress into my father's cleaning store. Although their siblings had known each other in their small town, my folks had been unaware of each other's existences until that day. Their families had come from the same village in Europe and then, oddly, settled in the same "New World" city of Paterson, New Jersey. It always struck me that there was a good fit with my Dad, Jack, being the oldest boy, the protective one in his family and my Mom, Lillian, the "baby" and the most vulnerable child in hers.

Despite some similarities, my parents' childhoods were very different from each other. Jack's family did well and quickly moved away to a nicer part of town. His memories of his youth were largely of having fun with his brothers, playing tennis and sharing laughs. Early on, Dad acquired an optimism that supported his belief in himself—he could accomplish almost anything if he set his mind to it. He spent the rest of his life pretty much proving himself right.

By contrast, my mother's siblings weren't playmates but older family members who, from her perspective, soon abandoned young Lil to a busy, widowed mother and a sense of loneliness and envy. She would tell me that the kids in school laughed at her for smelling of garlic and called her an orphan after her father died; she said that she never fit in. Young Lillian experienced a lot of shame that over her lifetime seemed to play a devastating part in her view of herself. Unlike Jack, Lillian often felt uncomfortable in social settings. Years later, when my mother dragged her young daughter to endless classes, she explained that she wanted me to be able to be comfortable in any setting.

Both my parents grew up watching their mothers work outside the home, which was unusual for that time. My Dad's mother was a passionate and engaged political activist with a newspaper column. The young Jack witnessed a woman's opinions being respected at home and out in the world; it's likely that this seeded his notion of how critically important a good education would be for his daughter.

My Mom's middle-aged mother was forced to go out and work when her husband died and her youngest child, Lil, was barely five. In order to make a living for the family, she took over her husband's candy store. Never having been taught to read or write, my grandmother had to invent a language and number system of her own to keep track of inventory and make change. That helped to explain my mother's oft-repeated advice that sounded revolutionary back in the 1950s: "Always have something to fall back on that you can do for yourself. Never rely totally on a man—not for your well-being or for your money."

The year was 1929 when Lillian and Jack graduated from high school. The Great Depression was sweeping the world and impacting the choices of that generation. My father bought a cleaning business from his brother-in-law despite having no prior background in the field. He did so partly to employ himself and his three younger brothers during troubling times and partly to rescue his brother-in-law's family from economic exhaustion.

When World War II came, Dad was excluded from the military because of a medical condition and he performed alternate service in a nearby airplane factory. Never one to sit around, during the six-minute break he had before the next valve would come down the assembly line, Jack started putting words to the music that the factory piped in. After World War II, Jack became a professional songwriter. I always loved that my father wrote songs for a living. I loved that he could be creative at work, since so many other parents seemed to have mundane jobs that they really didn't enjoy.

I was proud he'd chosen to do work he loved and that the product of that work, his songs, brought so much joy to himself, to others, and to me too. I also liked that, since he worked for himself and therefore had a great boss, he could design his own schedule. That afforded me lots of his attention and flexibility when it was needed. I was also thrilled that on occasion I could "help" Dad with his work. When I was in high school, endlessly practicing Beethoven's "Für Elise," Jack used my piano playing to inspire him to compose words to the piece, creating a popular song. At other times Dad requested my "teenage ears" to evaluate the currency of his lyrics. Years later I was struggling to decide whether I could change careers to become a psychotherapist and do work I hoped to love with no promises of future income. I recalled Dad's fearlessness in choosing to support his family with only royalties and no regular salary and used him as my inspiration.

My father was my mentor in creating the workable and optimistic philosophy that people should figure out what they want in life and then go for it. I would watch him discover a direction he wanted to go toward and then see him home in on making it happen. When the situation presented itself for my parents to have their version of the American Dream, a home of their own, Jack refused to let anything stand in the way. When the board of directors of the building turned down his application because Dad's livelihood writing songs would bring unwanted "entertainment business traffic," Jack brought in photos of my Mom and me, his quiet family, and convinced the naysayers they'd never regret admitting our family.

Mom's career path also began in 1929, but with some regret. She'd dreamed of becoming an English teacher but confessed she'd chosen to go to work over college as a reaction to her poor upbringing and the many financial challenges of the day. Having landed a good job in New York, seventeen-year-old Lilian had the funds to "do as she pleased" and to finally dress elegantly. As a result, she abandoned her dream and commuted daily to an office job in New York City.

Her persistence, another trait Mom shared with Dad, paid off. Lillian worked her way up the corporate ladder into an executive position in a large insurance company, a place few women had ever gone before. They also taught me by example that being persistent was a trait I'd want to adopt. Later in our POPcycle, when I had to delve into my parents' storage boxes, I unearthed my mother's high school yearbook where I saw her sweetly innocent face and her nickname: "Giggles"! I could hardly recall her ever laughing with complete abandon, and I had one of those moments most of us have from time to time when we realize how little we really know about our own folks, about the lives they lived before us and apart from us.

I missed not meeting Giggles or Mme. the Executive. The Lillian I knew worried a lot and was frequently temperamental and challenging with her perfectionism. Sadly, she often had difficulty feeling as much happiness as I'd have liked her to feel. But after we'd been doing POP for a while, she seemed to get that she'd never be abandoned and finally allowed herself to become more peaceful and happier—one of the many benefits I would see from taking on this challenge.

Who knows what attracts us to our mates? Jack had seen a sophisticated well-dressed beauty walk into one of his cleaning stores with her stained dress. "Who's the babe?" he'd asked his brothers. Lillian went home and told her nieces of the "perhaps too young man" who'd caught her notice, however briefly, with his attentiveness and caring ways.

Within several months, Jack had wooed, monopolized, and happily married Lillian. Together they left Paterson, New Jersey, their ten siblings, and their parents and "emigrated" across the state line to their chosen home in the Big Apple, New York City. There my folks rented an apartment on their own and started their life together, doing it "their way."

The years went by quickly as Jack wrote songs; Lillian attended to me, her husband, and the house; and I grew up. While I'd been on the move from New York to Boston to L.A., my parents had remained in the same location, the apartment that Jack had fought to buy. They gradually transitioned my former bedroom into the headquarters for Dad's international background music library business. As tapes and later CDs piled up where I'd formerly slept, it became less and less hospitable to sleep over. So, after I went off to college, I rarely went back to their home for very long.

My sights, like those of most young people, were pointed toward my future: the direction I was heading, and not behind me to the past or the places I'd come from. Perhaps like others, I didn't look back to notice that to some in our parents' generation, our choices seemed to be an abandonment or even a rejection of them. My parents had never expressed that thought to me directly, but until that Christmas visit, I'd never thought to ask either. As I looked at them now with new eyes that allowed me to see my parents' vulnerability differently, I wondered how Jack and Lillian had felt when their only child had moved so far away from them.

Whatever the rationale for leaving our first family, the fact is that emotional distances frequently accompany the physical distances between generations. Many very nice people in my generation would go for months, sometimes years, without seeing their parents during their twenties, thirties, forties, and fifties. Sometimes people got married, bought homes, joined the Peace Corps, and even had children that their parents had not yet met. Looking at Lillian and Jack in the apartment I'd grown up in, now so upside down, disarranged, and dusty, I considered that I too had actually gone sometimes for years without seeing my folks after moving across country. During that time, we stayed in touch with regular phone calls, and that had seemed to suffice.

All that had been so long ago, I thought, as I willed myself back into the present moment. I knew that, given all I was faced with, I would need to focus my attention on how we were going to navigate our interconnected futures, not ruminate too long on the past. Nonetheless, focusing was a challenge. Images and memories of years gone by kept appearing: the great times Mom and I had, staying with her family "in the country" when I was recovering from pneumonia at seven; Dad happily playing his latest song for his eager fan club president, me; the birthday when my beloved Aunt Miriam gave me my first pet, a wonderful kitten we'd named after a hit musical Dad's writing partner had on Broadway then.

I kept returning to the question: how would choosing to be there for Jack and Lillian in this new POP way change us and the relationships we'd had with each other up until now? I wondered how doing POP might alter the balance we'd been able to create in the dynamic of our family relationship but could find no template or any model to supply the answer. I was particularly concerned because my parents' needing help was showing up at the same time that I'd already committed to many other priorities as well. There were my patients, family, friends, and all the other things at home I'd said yes to. How could I include Mom and Dad on top of an already overfilled plate? And then again, how could I not include them?

I saw little, if anything, I could cross off my existing list of obligations. Whatever care or help I would be able to offer my parents would have to be added on to my current responsibilities. I didn't know yet where I would find the time or energy. I also had difficulty visualizing how caring for my parents would work on a practical basis. One question led to the next and the next.

Would I move back to New York and live with them? No. I knew immediately that wasn't going to be feasible for me as my practice and licenses were in California. Could they live in some senior home in New York? Could my parents come out to California to visit me as an interim solution? Would I find caregivers—one or more—for them in New York and then just jet home and leave them? How would I be able to supervise people working for my parents from such a long distance? Did they really need an official "caregiver," or would a domestic who could clean up the apartment and cook a meal now and then suffice? If Mom and Dad really needed to be looked after by a professional caregiver, how long could we expect that to last? And what might be the cost?

My head began to swim, but the questions kept coming at me. How many hours a day of care would they need? And how many days a week? Would I set up a plan to visit Mom and Dad in New York, say, once a month? Every month? Would visiting once a month be sufficient to accomplish all I might need to do for them? Or would visiting my parents monthly be too frequent, even feel oppressive to them? Would I need to have my aging folks move closer to me—now or in the future? The questions my mind came up with were endless. The answers were far less available.

Even when I thought I'd finished badgering myself with the unknown, I found I had still more unanswered questions. But this time, my questions were pointing to something more uplifting and less confusing. I found that, after a while, my mind was leading me to figure out the benefits that might accrue from taking on these new responsibilities.

Maybe I was being offered an unexpected invitation to show my generous and caring parents how much I appreciated all their sacrifices for me. Couldn't this be a chance to repay them for parenting me? Perhaps having this unique parenting experience with Jack and Lillian would help me be a better parent to my adult step-kids or their kids, my grandchildren. Wouldn't they all benefit from seeing me model caring for my Mom and Dad? Wouldn't my doing POP improve my skills as a psychotherapist as I helped others deal with their aging parents? I even wondered if caring for my parents would teach me how to be a more loving parent to the "inner child" in me.

As I started generating these answers, I felt some calm come over me. I recognized that eventually I would get my inquiries asked and answered—or maybe I wouldn't. I had long counseled others that when the time comes to make important decisions, we always have to operate with limited information or somewhat less than we'd like to know. Since it's impossible to know everything we'd like to know before deciding, at some point we must simply jump into choosing.

Choosing to do POP for my own parents became one of those leaps of faith for me. Put another way, the invitation to parent my parents evoked in me a humorous reference to *The Godfather*: for me, parenting Jack and Lillian was "an offer I could not refuse."

As I let the truth of that thought sink in, I noticed feeling an internal sense of peacefulness. My breathing became deeper, longer, and more energizing. I sensed a proper fit—there was rightness to my decision. I experienced a sense of wholeness in choosing to parent the people who'd parented me, even though I wasn't at all sure what that would look like. The Circle of Life was indeed completing itself.

I observed that I could choose to do POP in spite of having thoughts and feelings that were not always so loving or nice. There were times I was concerned, confused, and angry at my parents for having hidden their problems from me. In a flash, I had a recollection of when I'd been young and my parents had dissembled about various medical conditions they'd been diagnosed with for fear I'd become insecure knowing how old they were. As "late-in-life" parents, they had even lied to me about their ages until one night when they left me with a babysitter. I pulled down a book from their bookshelves that referenced Dad's musical compositions and age and learned the truth.

Accessing those memories of their concealing certain things allowed me to recall a long-forgotten family pattern that had persisted for years. However disturbing it was that they'd been hiding their conditions from me, remembering this behavior to be consistent with an old pattern actually comforted me. Back then, my parents had concealed things to protect me from what I didn't need to know or might have difficulty handling due to my childhood immaturity.

Although I didn't like what they were doing now, at least they were acting like the parents I'd known. As time evolved in our POPcycle, I often got sad, feeling that my parents were "disappearing." I would look for things that reminded me of how they used to be. Gazing at the people sitting in wheelchairs or lying in bed most of the day, sometimes I would search for the parents I used to know. Especially as they became frailer and weaker, I wanted to retain my memories of Jack and Lillian as vibrant, the way they'd been when I was young and the way they'd looked in photos before there'd even been a "me."

I was fortunate that Dad's personality stayed pretty much intact right through to the end of his life. He had a definite sweetness about him and an appreciative way that made it easy for anyone who attended to him. "Thank you, thank you, thank you," he'd say with a cute grin. Mom's progressive dementia made it harder to watch. I tried to make my way through the cloud that increasingly surrounded her. She would often be living in her past, hopelessly looking for her own mother to come visit her. Nonetheless, there were moments when I could still see the mother I remembered, even at ninety-five, and I particularly cherished the times when I could find her "still in there."

As a youngster, when I discovered they were concealing information, not only did I disagree with their model, but I also disliked the feelings it evoked in me. I felt excluded, condescended to, and resentful that others had held valuable information from me. I even determined that I would have been better served by seeing how my parents had resolved their challenges. I could have learned from their problem-solving skills rather than being blindsided by an illusion, believing that the problems didn't exist. Years later, although I could detect remnants of "protecting Jane" in their having hidden their need for my help, I saw it more clearly as my parents protecting themselves, mistakenly, from all that would happen—and did happen—once their true situation was revealed to me.

As a POParent, I would eventually concede some wisdom to my parents' point of view. There are moments in POParenting when it's appropriate to determine what is or isn't useful for an aging parent to know and, if they should be told, when. As Jack and Lillian got older, they became less coherent and more cognitively challenged. And as is often the case, my parents worried more as they aged than they had before, especially about little things. They also developed increased difficulty in processing information, and especially my mother had increased difficulty in hearing me altogether. This combination of factors led me to rethink my knee-jerk childhood conclusion that complete truthtelling is always best.

To make this point even clearer, there were times later on in our POPcycle when I would find myself not telling Mom or Dad certain things. If I suspected something would greatly upset them, ironically maybe now a medical condition of my own, I might not bring it up. At other times, if I could see that a topic was going be too complicated for them to comprehend, I might skip talking about it or censor something that previously I would have wanted to share with them.

In order to protect my aging parents, on rare occasions I would even lie to them. When they didn't wish me to supplement what their insurance company paid for their beloved caregiver, Florence, saying: "Don't pay any more for us," I failed to tell them that I did. Supplementing the caregiver was the best POParental choice. Occasionally, I'd say their insurance was paying for a treatment I felt was necessary when I was actually paying. I don't recommend dissembling as an everyday practice, but as we continued along our POP journey together, I found myself gaining an unexpected appreciation for some of my parents' earlier-in-life parenting decisions. But I'm getting ahead of myself again.

I discovered I could choose to do POP despite having had reactions and thoughts I was feeling ashamed of—like the denial

I'd been living with. How could I have imagined my parents would remain strong and living home alone forever? I knew the statistical likelihood that one out of two Americans over eighty-five would have some form of dementia, and my parents were each eighty-five. What had I been thinking or not thinking? Had I been my own patient, I would have counseled me, gently but definitely, to wake up from my delusions, since they held danger for all concerned. My denial had been effective in only one way—it left us all unprepared and in the middle of a crisis that could have been predicted. Maybe even prevented, too.

Sitting with my thoughts that day, I also uncovered a new feeling, an odd sense of power and influence I was pretty sure I didn't like. Maybe my parents were simply fearful of how much control I'd end up having over their lives and that was why they'd concealed recent events from me? That thought brought me no joy, I noticed. Having power over my parents' lives—or worse yet, responsibility for them—was still intimidating and overwhelming for me. I had difficulty owning it, but I knew what the truth was: increasingly over time, I would have to exercise my responsibilities—making decisions on their behalf and wielding my influence to get things accomplished for them, these new familial charges of mine.

It wasn't power that I wanted. Rather than being buoyed by my sway, I felt small and stressed by the pressures I was taking on—to organize a better or, at least healthier, life for two adult people. Planning a day for a ten-year-old child home from school on vacation is one thing, but planning a new life for my eighty-five-year-old parents took on awesome dimensions in my mind. What I really longed for was a magic wand so that my parents wouldn't be ill, in pain, or disabled—or die. But that was a momentary fantasy that came and went.

Knowing my parents, I knew they wouldn't be happy with the result, or with me, if I immediately started changing a lot in their lives or their home. I wasn't sure that my parents and I would agree on what a better life for them would look like. Nor was I certain what that was or how I could help create it for them. What

I did know was that some things would need to change whether my parents liked it or not. My inner voice was already sounding more POParental.

Time pressures were compounding my stress. Lillian and Jack were ill. I would need to return to California soon, and they'd barely been diagnosed—with what turned out to be pneumonias—let alone recovered. Was it irresponsible for me to leave them and go home? Was it irresponsible for me to stay with my parents, leaving things undone at home? It seemed like the POP version of the working mother conundrum: do I leave stuff undone at home or at work?

I didn't know how much I could accomplish for Mom and Dad before getting back to competing obligations at my home base. I didn't know when I could next afford to return to New York or how long I'd need to stay the next time. By "affording" to return, I wasn't simply referring to money for plane tickets or a hotel in New York City. I knew that each trip I made to attend to my folks meant leaving my practice, my family, and a host of responsibilities. How much time away could I afford, and how would my extensive travel schedule affect me?

I also wondered how much help I could be to my parents from a distance? Once I left New York, back in the pre-Skype/Face-Time days, I couldn't electronically or personally interview any geriatric care managers, caregivers, or domestic help. Once back in L.A., I couldn't go to my parents' doctors with them, nor could I ensure they follow the recommended treatments. I wondered if my parents would revert to their pattern of hiding things from me after I returned home. How much could I rely on paid people to follow through and report to me about Lillian and Jack's progress or compliance with doctor's orders?

Earlier when I'd felt guilty that I didn't want to "give up my life" to do POP, I'd found myself focusing on all I might lose. My concentration had been on what sorts of sacrifices choosing POP might create for me. Fortunately, my education proved helpful again, this time reminding me of something I knew but had forgotten. One definition of the word "sacrifice" is "something we make sacred," like an offering. Remembering this, I was able to revisit the notion of loss by asking myself: Was this reversal of our customary roles something I could choose to make sacred rather than fill it with struggle and loss?

All of a sudden, I saw an opening in my thinking. I'd found a way to look at this choice that moved me from potential losses to possible gains. I saw myself surfacing some different thoughts. What sorts of joy might doing POP generate? How much healing might all three of us find together now? How could doing POP expand my life? I didn't yet have the vision to see that, as with parenting children, the sacrifices of doing POP would ultimately pale in contrast to how much I would grow. I anticipated that the losses would be inevitable, but at this early point, I had no appreciation for how extensive my rewards would be.

In the quiet place where I decide important things and take the leap, what it came down to was this: POParenting Jack and Lillian was the right thing for me to do. I have no distinct memory of making a one-time, life-altering choice to parent my parents. It felt more like a gradual acceptance, making one choice at a time. I had no idea of precisely how, but I got that it would all work itself out somehow.

What I did choose that December day were our first POP steps in a journey of uncertain specificity or duration. However these unknowns turned out, parenting my parents was the right decision for me. It seemed that everything that had come before also now brought me here.

I would face many more POP decisions in the days ahead, almost too many. I intuitively recognized that taking those first POP steps represented a larger commitment to never leaving them alone—the people who'd raised me. With the choices I started making that December day, I knew I would remain aboard the POP ship with my parents, captaining it, in spite of rough seas and unforeseen weather, until it safely reached its final destination. That destination would culminate in their final breaths when Jack and, in turn, Lillian would no longer need me.

THEIR STORY—MOM

After all the hours I spent in psychotherapist offices and all the money Jack spent on the mission of my greater understanding and happiness, I should have noticed my denial more easily. But who among us wants to admit that at a certain age neither you nor your spouse can really make it without additional help from someone? Certainly I, who always prided myself on my ability to take excellent care of my family, my surroundings, and myself never expected to see such a day dawn. But it did more than dawn that Christmas Jane visited us from California—it kind of exploded.

She walked in on us unannounced after Jack had told her twice not to come. The place was pretty bad, so much dust and disorder. It had piled up and was just too much for me to handle on top of my exhaustion and coughing. I just couldn't function, and that itself had completely thrown me for a loop. Ordinarily I never get sick. And poor Jack could hardly keep up, trying to cook for us or order in and then clean up after. He just looked wiped out. I felt bad for him, but I was also scared: if he fell apart, who would take care of me?

As I look at it now, I think there had been some mutual denial going on between both Jane and us. Jane's been gone a long time. She moved away at seventeen to go to Wellesley and then stayed away, only returning home one summer to work in the city. We had to get used to her not being around and not coming back, but I'd long ago made my peace with that—with a little help from my first psychiatrist.

Jack and I managed well over the years, in spite of missing our only daughter. We were lucky enough to afford domestic help, but after a while, Jack gave up his office and we liked it nice and quiet at home. So, after a while we let our long-standing cleaning lady Louise go and just took care of the marketing, laundry, and dusting ourselves. It had worked fine until I got sick, I think. Maybe Jane would disagree with me about that.

She's a great arguer and an articulate advocate, Jane. A natural lawyer, my girl. But sometimes she gets a bit scary when she makes her mind up to do something or challenge you. And I don't want her to think she can come in here and tell us what to do and, frankly, I see a bit of a slippery slope here.

When my mother had her Parkinson's and couldn't care for herself at home, I remember how much my siblings and I fought over what to do with her. We all argued. There was no one in the family who could really nurse her at home, and I had Jane who was just a baby. I felt terrible, never wanting her to go to a nursing home. My big brothers won out, and she died there. I vowed that would never happen to me.

I do agree with this much: Jack and I need some help. But if we let her help with some things, how far will that go? I worry if Jane starts caring for us, where would that end? Not only that but she's very busy back home in L.A., and neither of us wants to interfere with that.

But I worry about how we'll manage everything if my sweet husband and I get sick again. Jane's getting people in to help right away, but in the long run, what will happen to us? Will we have to move? Will I end up like my mother?

Damn, this is overwhelming me. I wish I could keep this all a little better organized in my mind. I used to have such a remarkable memory. I think I need to lie down for a while.

YOUR STORY

Some of you feel you have no choice when it comes to parenting your parents. You are the only child or, simply, you love them. Others of you may feel you have few POP choices because of the mandates of the culture you grew up in. You may have heard since you were a child: "You must bring your aging parents into your home and care for them. This is what we do." Or you may have become the "designated" POParent by your siblings because you live close by and everyone else lives at a distance or, in some traditions, because you are the only daughter among sons.

I would like you to interrupt that type of reacting, believing that you have no choices, which could be called a form of "automatic" thinking. Anytime you feel you have only one choice in life you may be operating "on automatic" as contrasted with being and thinking in the moment. One of the most important things you will need as someone beginning to POParent is the willingness to think for yourself, based upon what is happening in the now.

Being your own thinker is often challenging, especially since so many "thoughts" are little more than automatic reactions to how you've been acculturated or trained to consider events. You have a wide range of choices in many circumstances and, in most instances, you have more options and solutions than you'd first considered.

Even if you can't imagine thinking the thought that you wouldn't invite your aging parents to live with you, you still have a host of choices to make about what and how you will help them. If you've already noticed your parents need some help, you will also need to consider: what kind of help do you think they will accept? What kind of help do you think they need? Knowing your parents, do you believe they will accept help from you? From whom else would your parents accept help? Who in your family is best suited to provide what your parents need—now and in the foreseeable future?

You have read how many different types of questions I asked myself during those initial days as I tried to surface answers about choosing POP and how I could reasonably "afford" to be there for them. When you need to make difficult or complicated decisions, ones that interlock with other decisions, asking yourself the right questions and then listening without censoring your answers is critical. In considering the questions that came up for me to grapple with, you have the benefit of my questions as well as all those you'll surface for yourself.

Certainly, one of the critical inquiries is this: Should you be the one who gives your parents POP help? That is, are your parents' requirements weightier than your ability to help or your actual willingness to do so? Simply because your parents are getting older and need some attention or care doesn't automatically mean you must be the one to POParent them. If you have siblings who live closer to your parents or more energetic adult grandchildren, or if one of your parents is much younger or healthier than the other, you may not need to take on the lead role in their POP. Maybe your role in POParenting will be better played out as a supporting one.

Did I think POP was a choice worth making? Of course I did, but it was a wise one and the best one for the three of us, given our circumstances and choices. Should everyone parent his or her own parents? No! Not in all cases.

Before any of you begins a POP journey, one caveat: POP is not for everyone! If your view of your family history is that your parent or parents abandoned you, abused you, neglected or betrayed you, and you are still carrying emotional or physical scars to show it, perhaps you should stop right here. At the least, I recommend you seek further advice from a professional—a religious or mental health counselor or a certified POP Family Coach—before you undertake to do POP.

In certain circumstances, both you and your parents would be better off were the POP job turned over to others—siblings, professionals, neighbors, others. If your instinct tells you there are dangerous waters ahead in doing POP, get some sage advice and consider it carefully. You need to listen carefully to yourself as well as contemplate the advice you receive from those you've sought to counsel you. Parenting isn't for the fainthearted and POParenting is hardly an exception to that rule. If you're feeling guilt or confusion associated with parenting your parents—or not doing POP—you and they are likely to benefit from your getting some professional counseling beforehand. If you reflect on how casual some of us were about choosing parenthood when we were young, you'll see some of the benefits of carefully considering the POParental choice before you commit to it.

Some of you already have decided you're going to choose—or have already chosen to do POP. And although you think you should act in a loving and kind way, you may discover you are still filled with unspoken, even unconscious anger or unresolved bitterness toward your family. Doing this job and being around your parents more often may kick up long-forgotten memories and feelings, some of which may not be desirable. Again, this would be a good time to seek a little help from an expert, someone wise and equipped to help you heal unwanted feelings—before you get too deeply involved with POP. As you will soon discover, doing POP while you're still harboring those types of feelings is not optimal.

Why is POParenting out of obligation or with resentment a tough go? Caring for your elderly loved ones requires a lot of consistency and follow-through, just like parenting your children did. If you're stewing inside while you're trying to act caringly, that might emerge in ways that further damage your aging parents or the new relationship you're aiming to build with them.

Have you started down an irretrievable path to becoming your parent's parent just because you agreed to make a few phone calls for your mother or volunteered to balance her bank statements? No. Can't you just do a few odd jobs for your aging folks when you're available without having to start a whole POP relationship? Yes, you can.

If you make those calls or do some odd jobs, are you then obligated to go to all your parents' doctor appointments or move them into your home? No, you're not. You'll only be making one POP choice at a time. You should make only the commitments that you're willing to follow through to their completion. And your follow-through involves checking in: how is your recent POP decision actually working out? Are the results as you intended? Is that commitment working well for your parents and for you?

Sometimes it's hard while doing POP to "keep good boundaries," a term that therapists use to talk about healthy emotional distances we place between others and us. Often doing POP intrudes on your comfortable or traditional boundaries with your parents. These shifts in your long-held roles may end up challenging you in ways you can't expect. You have a new kind of power over your parents. They may be leaning on you, even literally, as you used to need to lean on them. You're making important choices for them, like they used to do for you when you were a child. You may now be deciding where they'll live, who'll care for them, or when they'll go to senior day care.

How do you keep good boundaries when you're feeling so many emotions—literally looking down on your parents in their wheelchairs, shouting at them so they can hear you or helping them transfer into your car's backseat like you did with your infants? You will need to take good care of yourself through this process. Take some time to find out what's okay with you and what doesn't feel right and then learn to articulate these boundaries with kindness.

Fortunately, you don't do POP all at once, and that makes having all these feelings far more manageable. You only can do one POP thing at a time. You take one POP step before you take another. One POP decision will lead you to the next step. Things may feel out of our control when you're doing POP, and retaining a sense of calm is part of your new challenge.

You will want to ask yourself: will you be there, if your POP journey lasts for a decade or longer? The average number of years people parent parents is increasing, as we are all living longer. Many gerontologists believe that people who are now fifty may spend at least eighteen years caring for their aging parents, given the increasing longevity of seniors and other factors. Your POP years may even exceed your child-rearing ones. Entering the POP journey with the notion that it will be short and sweet will leave you ill prepared for the realities of twenty-first-century longevity, medicine, and so much more.

You stand the best chance of having a satisfying and successful POP experience if you can be there for your parents because you want to be and you're prepared to make the commitment to do POP from that perspective. Some of you may also have thoughts that since your parents parented you, you "should" do the same for them. Obligation is a motivator for many, as is guilt, although neither is optimal here. It will be very helpful to you in developing your POP relationship if you can manage to shift your perspective from obligation/guilt to something more positive, like gratitude and compassion. See if you can focus on what you appreciate about your parents. Or if that doesn't work right now, try focusing your gratitude on your being healthy and strong enough to POParent them.

We do this POP job best if we're clear that we have chosen to go on this journey. Do I think POP is the right choice? For most people, my answer is a resounding "*Yes!*" The sooner you discover the breadth of your parents' needs and who and what can meet those needs, the sooner you can take responsibility for making your POP choices based upon your own boundaries and your life situation.

It is likely to be getting clearer that your decision to do POP will have long-term effects, planned and unplanned, on your life and the lives of everyone around you. Although the decision to POParent is yours alone, I strongly recommend you also talk in detail with those your choice will impact the most—your spouse, business partner, or children who still live with you. POParenting may offer most of you an inspiring life change but no choice is right for everyone. You must search your own heart and mind and then act in concert with them.

If you do choose to invest yourself in POP, be wary to not extend yourself beyond your own doable limits. Sometimes it gets hard for us caring POParents to know where those limits are or to ask for help when, or better yet before, we've reached them. You will wear yourself ragged and be of little good if you overpromise and then can't live up to what you've offered. It's critical that while you're POParenting you learn to know when enough is enough for you, too. Your parents may need to hear you say, "That's enough for me for today," when it truly is. You can't do POP well and for a long time unless you also pay attention to caring for yourself and becoming your own advocate. That theme will recur as we do this POParenting together.

Most of your aging parents truly appreciate what you're doing for them, even if it isn't perfect and even if they complain. Your parents really do feel safer once you've intervened, and they are grateful. Your parents are also proud of you for choosing to parent them. As you begin to do POP, don't be surprised to notice that your parents are feeling good about how they raised you and how that contributed to your so thoughtfully giving back to them. Although POP can seem to be a gift from you to your aging parents, it may be that you're receiving the bigger gift.

Are you ready?

3

ENTERING POP IN THE MIDDLE OF A CRISIS

MY STORY

That morning, showing up on their doorstep when I was told not to, was the unofficial commencement of POP, Wolf Style. Viewed from the perspective of how our parent-child relationship had been up until that morning, going to my parents' apartment when I'd specifically been told to stay away was an act of defiance. But in our newly developing dynamic, arriving there unexpectedly and against my father's expressed wishes was an act of responsible POParenting. It felt like it was my first.

According to researchers, when we're trying out new behavior, repetition makes us more comfortable. POP was no exception in the sense that I did get more relaxed with certain "intrusive" POP activities as time wore on. But even then, I was never truly at ease when POParenting looked like it involved defying Mom or Dad's stated requests.

Worse yet were those exceptional times when I'd have to verbally "discipline" them for something or intercede to stop Mom from hitting Dad. At those times, they acted just like kids! POP would repeatedly make demands on me that were so unexpected that they felt almost unnatural. My way of responding would be to reach into a place deep inside of me—a place of courage, internal knowing, and extraordinary compassion—just to discover how to act as the good parent to my parents. Although my parents had resembled the other people in the restaurant that night, for the first time they'd also reminded me of young children in their slow and deliberate way of walking and thinking. I realized that I might have to think about my parents differently and sometimes behave differently toward them.

When Dad opened the door, there were two still unfamiliar people standing in front of me in their faded pajamas. "I told you not to come. What are you doing here? Why are you here?" he repeated, as if his questions made any sense.

"I'm here, Dad, because there's something very wrong with Mom and with you and—now that I see it, with the state of your apartment as well. I'm here out of love and because I want to help you. I get that you don't want me to know all that's happening, but you need some assistance and I'm here now," I said. I was trying out my calmest, sweetest, and best newly minted POParental tone. "Please let me help you!" I offered, even more softly. I watched as my Dad just kind of melted in front of me. In spite of his gruff tone and unwelcoming greeting, he seemed—not far from the surface—to be glad I had come.

Mom, however, wasn't doing a lot of "melting," nor was she capable of lucid conversation or logical thinking. Intermittently, her attitude was belligerent, and she was disoriented. She seemed highly anxious and hypervigilant, as if something were about to be taken away from her, but she also seemed too confused to recall what that was.

My first phone calls were to each of their physicians. My parents needed medical care—today. I wanted them to be seen by their own physicians, not by some emergency room person who knew nothing of their histories. They had two different internists, and I was able to make appointments for each of them for a "quick visit" that day. Dad's doctor diagnosed pneumonia, gave him some antibiotics, told me to make sure he got ample rest and fluids, and suggested that recuperating at home would be healthier than in the hospital. But I was also informed that, should he stay at home, my overworked daddy would need an attendant to care for him twenty-four hours a day while he was recovering.

Mom's doctor was concerned about the pneumonia she, too, had contracted. He felt Lillian needed immediate hospitalization, but by now it was New Year's Eve and New York was being buried under a snowy blizzard. Her physician worried that the emergency rooms would soon be overrun. He reasoned Mom would gain admission faster into nearby Mt. Sinai Hospital if a specialist, a psychiatrist, referred her there rather than if he, a generalist, did so or if we just walked in. I didn't really understand why that would make for a speedier entrance process, but I took his recommendation: my first of many POP discoveries about how the experts could help work the system to my parents' benefit.

Leaving his office, we found that the snowstorm made hailing a cab a chore in itself, but getting my parents into and out of the cab provided an even harder challenge. We must have made quite the spectacle on the streets of Manhattan's Upper East Side. Mom again was looking ragtag and disoriented. When I tried to extract her from the cab, it probably looked like I was dragging out a dead body.

Then I tried to maneuver Dad out of the taxi and into the cold. He was shaking and seemed off-balance as he stepped onto the slippery street. I was oddly grateful, in that moment, for Dad's senile osteoporosis, a condition that reduces bone mass, since he now was closer to five eight than his original six-foot frame. But even with his loss of height, I was still unable to hold him up. He collapsed to the street and momentarily lay in a pile in the snow. Getting him to his feet and walking them both into the building and then down the short corridor from the elevator took a good twenty minutes. It seemed more like a bad twenty hours.

Next, I took my mother to a psychiatrist, as recommended, for a referral to get into Mt. Sinai. I had the pleasure over the following years of doing POP to encounter some truly extraordinary individuals who helped me parent my parents in so many different ways. There were caregivers, nurses, physical therapists, social workers, doctors, dentists, lawyers, and neighbors—so many kind and truly caring people that I came to treasure along the way. Unfortunately, the psychiatrist who saw my mother that afternoon was not such a man. He literally screamed at me for bringing her to him. "How could you even consider bringing such a sick woman to my office?" he demanded to know. No help here, we'd be left with the last resort, going to the ER.

As I was helping my folks back into their mufflers, mittens, and boots as we were leaving the psychiatrist's office, my thoughts went back to my childhood and I recalled their having dressed me into my mufflers, mittens, and boots in order to protect me from other New York winters. Now I made sure they were warmly wrapped up and protected as we all headed back downstairs for our next transportation experience. By the time I finished POP ten years later, I couldn't recall a single holiday when I hadn't been in the ER with one or both of my parents. This New Year's Eve was simply the first.

It was also that night that Lillian gave me the idea to name what I was beginning to do "Parenting Our Parents." After waiting the expected number of hours, Mom, Dad, and I were finally sitting in a cubicle with the ER nurse. When we found out that my Mom was only getting 76 percent of her oxygen, her bizarre behavior made sense. The reason she'd been acting psychotic or like someone in the late stages of Alzheimer's was due to oxygen depletion from her pneumonia. Lillian couldn't think straight, quite literally, with that small amount of oxygen going to her brain.

But sitting there in front of the nurse, even before anyone could give her any additional oxygen, Mom appeared to have miraculously transformed herself into a highly intelligent and cognizant woman. Asked if she knew her name, Lillian carefully spelled out her full name including her maiden name. "Address?" Lillian was perfect, down to her apartment number and the zip code, thank you. What happened to the irrational woman we'd been dealing with earlier today? Previously she'd been biting and scratching, but now she was responding with crisp precision to the nurse's questions.

All of a sudden, I got it! When I was young, Mom had often repeated one of her scariest fears to me: being "locked up" in a nursing home. Apparently back in the 1940s my grandmother had suffered from advanced Parkinson's disease and, over Lillian's objections, the older siblings had placed their mother in a nursing home. Mom had always been afraid that she too, would be "locked up" someday by her family. I suspected that my mother's survival instincts kicked in to her oxygen-deprived brain and provided her those precise answers in order to guarantee her liberty. But I was totally unprepared for what followed next.

Seeking to discover whether the patient was oriented, the nurse asked: "Who brought you to the hospital tonight, Lillian?" With the defiant look of a six-year-old, my Mom wheeled around in the cubicle, screwed up her face and pointed directly at me: "*My mother did!*" I saw it in a flash: I was about to become my own mother's mom. What I was facing ahead would be parenting my parents!

I initially thought that her response was attributable to the oxygen depletion. However, upon further reflection, I realized that her "accusation" and attribution of mothering to me was oddly prescient. I was becoming her mother in the most basic and essential way, by acting to protect her. Perhaps I was even acting like the mother she wished she still had.

No matter what Lillian was thinking at that moment, she'd given me another name for what was beginning, and she was uncannily on point. I was now the one becoming her parent, her new POParent. I was there in the ER that night as I would be there for her over the next ten years in the role of her POP Mom.

When they finally admitted Mom into the hospital for her pneumonia that evening, Dad also was told for the first time that his beloved bride was suffering with dementia. He learned that her illness, which they called Alzheimer's, would become far more serious progressively and, ultimately, he wouldn't be able to handle it by himself. As a result, Dad came to recognize that together we would have to get more help for Mom and for him, too. Knowing he wouldn't be alone on this journey, for the first time on this whole visit my father looked me directly in the eye and deeply exhaled.

Later, after the initial crisis, and during much of the earlier stages of POP, I was able—and I wanted—to involve my parents in most of the POP decisions. But in those first days and nights, neither parent was physically or emotionally able to participate in those decisions, as is often the case when we show up in the middle of a POP crisis. When I brought Dad back from the ER and left him with this news and at home without Mom for the first time in decades, he was very quiet. I wondered how he truly felt, but he wasn't one to talk a lot about such things.

Now that I had the time to survey their scene more carefully, I too felt overwhelmed. It was exhausting to look at the myriad of things ahead I would need to "fix." I also felt profoundly alone. This feeling was something different, deeper than I'd known before. I was in the most populated city in the world, or one of them. I had a good support system, but I didn't know how to get support for these feelings I was having. My sense of isolation, the overwhelmingly heavy responsibility, a fear of messing up and doing POP wrong were some of the emotions that drifted through me. I didn't want any of those feelings, but I recognized them as authentic. As I look back on it now, I think I was "processing," getting ready to accept the responsibilities of doing POP.

Choosing to become a parent is an awesome choice. Choosing to parent the people who raised me and now were old and needing me seemed nothing less than mind-blowing—a full-blown role reversal! It also triggered other feelings long forgotten—like the burden I'd felt as an only child to older parents, wanting to be sure I'd do well enough to make up for other children my parents wouldn't ever have—or the feelings that had led me to create the only child's proverbial imaginary friend.

Early on in life, I'd learned how to convert the aloneness of being an only child and my sense of responsibility for that into more useful qualities, seeding self-reliance, resourcefulness, and an ability to get on easily with grown-ups. Now, in order to do this new POP job well, I'd need to marshal all the skills I'd ever developed and apply all the education I'd ever had. Unfortunately, when I began parenting Lillian and Jack, there was nothing I could find to really guide me through this stage of life, this role reversal. Nothing at all.

Recall that there were no blogs then on aging parents, no POP-arenting magazines offering me any calming advice, no one around to coach me. There was no guidance to show me how to work my way through the changes. Back then, there wasn't even anyone thinking in terms of POP or developing the notion of a POPcycle, seeing it as a time for healing, expanding, even exchanging our roles with our parents. I felt like a geriatric pioneer, cutting brush and laying trails for those who would follow with their similar needs for POP help.

We were fortunate in my family that I had a legal background even more extensive than my geriatric experience. Knowing the law allowed me to be comfortable looking over their legal and financial documents, talking to their doctors, lawyers, and accountants. I used those analytic skills and found that I was empowered when I could put my attention on the things that were known instead of the many unknown, out-of-control things.

Of course, not everyone POParenting can offer their parents the particular advantages that my education and training afforded Lillian and Jack. Nonetheless, everyone doing POP will bring his or her own unique expertise, talents, and background to the POP experience. And now you have the added advantages of my POP trail to follow from reading this book and the remarkable contributions other POParents are making on the POP website (http://www.ParentingOurParents.org).

But I couldn't figure out how much help or even what kind of help my folks would need until I had a complete picture of where Jack and Lillian were at physically, cognitively, financially, legally, and spiritually. My parents would only be able to provide a relatively small amount of that data if they were like most of my older patients. Their ability to recall recent events was less sharp than their long-term memories. I'd need other sources of information from both people and records to verify what they told me and to learn more.

No matter one's professional expertise and no matter whether one has siblings or is an only child, no one can adequately and satisfyingly care for aging parents as a one-person band. I knew I would need to start forming a team of people, my TEAM POP. These are the people I would rely on to both help me make POP decisions and also to help me carry them out.

I'd need someone on my team who could act like my eyes and ears for the majority of the time when I was not there in New York, someone who possessed a good set of local contacts for the things my parents would need over the next few days, weeks, and months ahead. What I wanted was a mature professional who could reliably check up on Lillian and Jack on some kind of a regular basis, although I didn't yet know how often that might be. What I needed was a geriatric care manager (GCM), a professional whose job description involves doing all of that for families like mine.

To find a GCM to help us, I started by contacting some of my lawyer friends who practiced geriatric law in New York. I also remembered that, during a recent reunion, some of my New York high school friends had talked of hiring caregiving help for their parents. I went through my memory bank and Rolodex resources that were around before Google was invented to locate well-respected GCMs.

Wasting no time, as I had none to waste, I set several appointments for the following day. Then I sat down to write out questions I thought I'd need to have answered to hire a good GCM. I asked myself: what would someone interested in working for my family in the GCM job want to know about my parents and, from the other side, what would I want to know about the GCM?

I tried to figure out how much information I should supply to the GCM applicants. Were I to prepare an outsider to be my eyes and ears, how much of my family's usual dictum of "let's keep family matters private" would I have to ignore? Many in my parents' generation shared similar beliefs that no one outside the family should know "private matters," but I recognized that approach might be highly misplaced here during POP. Should I tell a GCM during an interview that my mother has a history of being difficult or not?

By doing research and initiating action, I avoided sitting around and "marinating." With little time for contemplation, I decided my best course was to use my energies to take action and not engage in worrying or trying to figure it all out in advance. I discerned that I'd be forced to figure many things out as I went along and, somehow, that would have to be all right. Doing the research helped me make better decisions and taking action supported my ability to feel energized and gain confidence, part of the recipe for POP relief.

Over the course of the next day, I interviewed all the GCMs on my list, checked their references, and hired the one who seemed the best fit for Mom and Dad. I hoped my choice would be okay, and having made it, I actually felt relieved. Taking these steps helped a lot. It felt good that I was beginning to create some order, and I liked the reassurance the GCM gave me that when I left town, some of the POP burdens would be shared with an experienced professional.

When the GCM arrived to start work the following day, I was almost elated. It was remarkably comforting to have her calmness and, since she did this every day, to feel we were normal and like other POP families. I'd been impressed with the GCM's list of possible workers, and clearly we needed someone to clean the apartment from top to bottom. I followed all the ideas our GCM recommended that first day. She not only found us a cleaning woman but when we needed new equipment (since Mom's vacuum was literally scotch-taped together) the GCM knew where to go and how to get things delivered quickly.

Our GCM also had a long list of possible caregiving candidates, and I needed to hire several, since my father required round-the-clock nursing. His doctor had insisted on that as the trade-off for not hospitalizing him. The GCM asked me to fully "explain" each of my parents so she could best match her candidates with their personalities.

I then interviewed many women for the initial caregiver positions and even a few men. I understood that even after Mom returned from the hospital, she would need help too. I hoped the daytime caregiver I saw as best for Dad could also help with Mom. I anticipated that any caregiver working with Lillian would need extra patience and a good layer of thick skin. As far as I could see ahead, which wasn't very far, both my parents would need someone with them for a good portion of their day, perhaps for a long time.

You can imagine that I had misgivings about hiring anyone to help with my parents. Would anyone be as careful or caring with them as I might be? Would my parents feel safe with strangers staying in their apartment when they were sleeping? Would these caregivers be reliable to get them healthy food, buy him the right socks, and take them both to the doctors' appointments that I clearly couldn't attend?

I knew from the beginning that I was unwilling to give up my work and uproot my life by moving back to New York City. As a result, I had to find a team of people I could rely on. I needed to find a balance where I wouldn't be micromanaging everyone but could still have the confidence that I was properly informed and attending to my parents' well-being.

I would have to learn to depend on people who were not family to act as family members would for each other. I would need to set standards, whatever they might be, and provide my aging parents adequate protection from any sort of abuse or neglect. Would receiving regular reports be sufficient? How often would I want to personally visit and see what was happening? With new people in their apartment, how would I safeguard their valuables? I could see that the GCM would be overseeing the caregivers, but I also understood that I would need to have responsibility for everyone, including the GCM.

Our family was blessed when we found Florence. She came to us as the GCM's brilliant recommendation to be Dad's daytime caregiver. Initially when he was recovering from the pneumonia and exhaustion, Dad needed 24/7 help and Florence was hired as the day person. For a time, he needed three shifts of people doing eight-hour shifts for full-time caregiving but it was Florence who was there through the waking portions of Dad's day. I could see immediately that Florence would be a godsend. Implausibly, she'd previously worked for another family in our building, so she even knew the apartment staff, how to get around the building, and our neighborhood, all on day one.

When Mom returned, Florence stayed on. She took care of both my parents through some grim days and nights, as you'll read more about soon. Intuitively, she seemed to know how to treat both Jack and Lillian: how much kindness or strictness to show and how much warmth or distance. I particularly valued her consistency, grace, and patience—qualities anyone should seek out in a prospective caregiver.

Any professional caregiver for aging parents puts up with all that goes on over the course of years in a family's life: parents living in pain; people getting grumpy "without reason"; childish behavior and demands. I also felt very fortunate to have someone begin at the POP beginning and to work consistently with them until I brought them to California from New York. That continuity helped me feel safer, especially when I was at such a distance from them.

I'll get to that down the POP journey a ways, but what I learned those very first days was that my caring for Lillian and Jack would have to be a hands-on job. I could assign tasks to others but, in the end, it would be I who would need to be their POParent. And since I was going to stay in California and they apparently would be staying in New York, I would need to discover how to make this arrangement work.

YOUR STORY

You too may need to get some help for your parents, both for your own well-being and for theirs. You may see getting additional help as particularly valid if you've found yourself in the middle of some POParental crisis and have discovered that there are things you need to "repair" that led to the crisis, as well as strategic, long-term POPlanning to do for what lies ahead.

For most of us, neither the birth of our children nor the discovery that our aging parents need our help is ordinarily planned optimally. Undoubtedly you would prefer to have some of the "conversations" and initiate some POPlans before any crisis occurs, and maybe that is still an option for you. I certainly hope so.

But if you have an elderly loved one in your life, in all likelihood—at some point—that loved one will become seriously ill, take a fall and break a hip, need you on their Advance Health Directive form, or require grab bars installed in the bathroom yesterday! As you can see, you too will need a TEAM POP to help you and your parents do POP. You'll want to begin getting the members together *before* a crisis begins.

To be complete, a good POPlan should include how you will take care of yourself as well as your parents, even what should happen in the event you predecease them. Taking care of yourself may offer unique challenges. POParenting may require you to give up doing some things you've cherished. Traveling, seeing friends often, or even doing work you've loved may take a backseat for a while. You will need the discipline of prioritizing what's most important for all concerned. Taking care of your parents may cause your social life to dwindle, and that may continue for quite some time.

The aging loved ones you're attending to may well outlive you! The people doing POP and/or family caregiving frequently find they cut back on doing the things they used to do that provided them relaxation and social support. They attend church less often and see acquaintances less frequently. Even more significantly, if you're a family caregiver, you may need to reduce your hours at work or cease your employment altogether. If you reduce your hours to less than twenty per week, you may no longer be eligible for certain benefits. You may not even be able to afford health insurance at the very time you're likely to need it the most.

Others of you will need to find paid help to supplement your family caregiving when you're not there. The family member most qualified to recruit, interview, and hire professional help for your parents will hopefully be available to do so. Having someone who lives close to your parents will make your job of finding caregivers and other workers easier. But you may be equally able to locate a GCM, employment services, or in-home caregiving teams online. Today you can interview potential workers via Skype or FaceTime and watch them interact with you and other family members, wherever you all are located. You can use these modern methods whether you're POParenting long distance or locally and whether they've come recommended by your parents' doctors, the insurance company's registry, or other POParents you've met on the POP website.

Once you've hired some caregiving help, overseeing them may take a variety of forms, and as usual in POP, one size does not fit all. Your family may want to regularly review written or verbal reports from anyone helping your parents, like you did with those who taught or took care of your children. If you have siblings, you may assign reviewing those reports to the most qualified one to respond appropriately. Others may adopt a practice that has been simplified by the internet: rather than sending reports to only one sibling who will be the chief communicator, all of you can be placed on a distribution list—siblings, spouses, or other intimates—and receive emails with those reports.

If you or a family friend can drop in on your aging parents to check on them and their caregiver unexpectedly, you might find that very instructive. Some people even get the equivalent of nanny cameras secretly installed in their parents' homes to watch those caring for their senior loved ones, and they can receive such videos in real time anywhere in the world. Utilizing twenty-first-century communication tools, you and your TEAM POP can determine the amount of safety you feel is necessary and the amount of watchfulness you can afford.

If you have paid help in your parents' home, you will want to be appropriate about securing and/or removing their valuables. Often family members give caregivers access to their parents' residence, checkbooks, credit card data, and computers in order that they can be helpful. Nonetheless, do not overlook the fact that your parents' jewelry, art, cash, identity items, checkbooks, negotiable instruments, and even their stamp collections could be temptations. And remember that senior parents often spend much time sleeping and that may leave such items vulnerable to theft or to being misplaced. If these types of things have been left around at your folks' home, it would be wise to consider storing them somewhere safer. You'll also want to avoid giving out unnecessary identifying information, computer passwords, and anything that might allow access to your parents' financial accounts unless you consider it critical that your parents' aides know this information. In my experience, it rarely is necessary to share such confidential information.

Again, fellow POParents, remember to trust yourself. You will need to listen to yourself! If you don't have a good feeling about potential employees who will have your parents' minds, bodies, and spirits under their care, do not hire them. Legally and emotionally speaking, it's always easier not to hire someone than it is to let him or her go after there's a problem.

4

LEARNING MORE THAN WE WANTED TO KNOW

Our Parents' Financial, Health, Legal, Spiritual, and Other Issues

MY STORY

I made a series of trips to New York that first year I was POParenting Lillian and Jack. Much of my agenda during those visits was to gather information I would need to help them feel and become safer, now that I was "on board." Like most things POP, it took longer than I'd anticipated to get the information from my folks and then to follow through with whatever else was needed.

When I arrived at their apartment on any day of such inquiry, I'd immediately be struck by the fact that my parents did everything substantially slower than I did. They thought slower, moved slower, decided things slower than most people my age did. Their experience of time and ability to focus were also different from mine. I saw that I'd need to take lots of deep breaths and literally slow down so that the sheer force of my energy and the speed with which I ordinarily operated didn't overwhelm my parents.

I would show up in the morning, ready to get down to it but my parents might or might not be ready for me or for the next task on my list. I was learning from my parents, just as we learn from our children how to most effectively parent them. I soon discovered I'd need to speak more slowly, perhaps with more volume, to repeat myself, to make sure they understood what I was asking. Most of all, I'd have to become more patient. That couldn't be bad.

My ultimate goal in gathering all this information was to create additional security for my declining parents, whether that was physical, legal, or financial security. Making them safe seemed relatively straightforward when I was having grab bars installed in their bathrooms. It wasn't always so easy to figure out other ways to keep them safe.

Making my parents safe required me to review each document and decision, one at a time. It also involved asking them endless questions, prying through years of well-worn papers, and generally intruding into their lives. I had not lived with my parents in over thirty years and, even with me, my parents were private people. Whenever they'd gone to others instead of asking for my legal advice over the years, I'd tried not to take it personally. Given what I was unearthing in some of their documents, I could see that keeping me uninformed had not been their best choice.

My asking them questions, digging up old memories, reviewing their past decisions, and opening tens of boxes full of papers was bound to be emotionally triggering for all of us. I saw how Mom's cognitive limitations were adding to her emotional challenges. She would try to maintain her focus and to recall answers, or she would compensate by making up an answer, revealing the limitations she was all the while trying to hide from herself and me.

Over time, the process got a little easier. But the first day of doing this inquiry was one of the hardest for me. There would be other very demanding days to come—like their accidents leading to hospitalizations or the day I put Dad on hospice or when I couldn't find a mental facility that would accept Mom. But in the Wolf family saga, the toughest days seemed to be when one of my parents interpreted an event as symbolizing the loss of control over life. Usually that resulted in a panicky parent, and almost always that was Mom.

Lillian turned out to be much tougher to POParent than Jack. During her twenties, she'd occupied important positions that demanded great organizational skill, and she was naturally obsessive. As a result, she'd become the "designated domestic organizer" at our house. Mom's bedroom closet was the repository for their most important records. She came from the rubber-band school of organizing. That is, papers were bound together by rubber bands, some worn and stretched out, and others pristine. I'd ask, "How much do you and Dad receive from Social Security each month?" Mom would direct me first to the closet, then to a box, and then to the particular packet of papers. I'd have to bring it out and, in front of her, unwrap the rubber band, read the papers, and take any notes I needed. Then she needed me to wrap the rubber band around the packet of papers again and return them to the box in the closet before returning to her for my next inquiry. We would have to go through this process for each question I posed.

When it felt to Lillian like her whole life was swirling out of her control, she did what most people do when they feel helpless. She drew a line in the sand: *No one messes with my rubber band system!* It went this way for hours and hours. On the outside, I was the most patient person ever, but on the inside, I was a mess. I tried to be kind and understanding. I even introduced self-talk and thought about how challenging it must have been parenting me. But as soon as I could "safely" leave that first day of questioning them, I ran the short block to a cafe, where I focused exclusively on a frosty margarita, actually several.

The problem really was with me, not Mom, I soon saw. She'd been well organized her whole life, and my being there now, intruding on her privacy and upsetting her system with my demands must have deeply upset her and compromised her sense of order and control. As I mulled over the thought that she wasn't just trying to be difficult, I was able to muster more understanding. And more patience.

During January and February of 1998, the bitterest of months in the Northeast, I made four brief visits to New York, flying back and forth across our wide, three-time-zoned continent to be there for my parents. I remember feeling dislocated on both coasts. Even before leaving home for one of those body-bruising three- or four-day trips, I would spend hours rescheduling my patient appointments and other events. I had to book travel and even lodging, since it had become clear I couldn't stay in my parents' overcrowded and cluttered space.

On those occasions I would leave home early in the Pacific morning when it was still dark, hoping the taxi horn didn't wake my neighbors. By the time I would arrive in New York, it would be dark, and I would be tired, achy from the plane ride, and pretty useless. Although the airlines call it a five-and-a-half-hour flight, it never took me less than nine hours to go between my L.A. home and my hotel in the Big Apple. I also had decided to delay my own much-needed foot surgery while taking care of this phase of POP-arenting. Thus, I had to endure painful hikes down long airport corridors, dragging my carry-on and occasionally limping, which didn't make my treks any easier. By the fourth trip, I began to be a bit concerned for my own well-being. I wasn't getting any young-er, either. I was also feeling "dislocated" mentally, pulled in many different directions, as new parents sometimes describe.

I had liked my life before, and even though I'd made the choice to do POP, I was still reluctant to fully accept the bicoastal life and the other adaptations I had to make. One of the most helpful insights I had about my own resistance during this part of our POPcycle was this: It wasn't useful to bemoan the loss of "my life"; it was better to embrace my expanding into a bigger life, which included POP. "My life" and even my view of myself needed to be large enough to include Jack and Lillian as a priority. Sometimes they were the greatest priority. In making these trips to POParent them, I was beginning to prioritize my parents' needs over my patients' needs.

I wondered about the long-term effects POParenting Jack and Lillian would have on my new practice, my income, my psyche, and other parts of my life. Only on occasion would I allow myself to muse upon the unknown unknowns. Most of the time, having made the POP commitment, I turned to my next step and kept on going. There was always so much to do.

YOUR STORY

You too, will have to get past whatever initial reluctance you might have to ask your parents *the* most personal of questions. If you have siblings, this is a perfect time to divide up different parts of the POP "inquiry" job. Each of you can take charge of one or two areas. If you have some delicacy about money but your sister Sally, the accountant, has none, she's likely the better one to get your parents' answers about their investments, income, and expenditures and, later, to locate, organize, and evaluate their financial issues.

If Sally is unavailable, has long-standing emotional problems with your parents, lives abroad or for some other good reason, is not the optimal choice to lead that inquiry, you may need to use

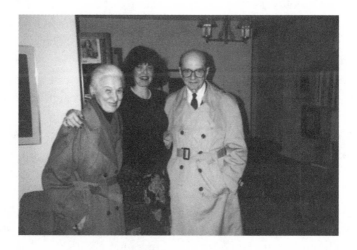

Figure 4.1. We're all getting shorter too.

slightly different approaches. Your parents may have forgotten much, and that can't feel good to them, or you. Your reminding them of things from their past might result in sadness or even giggling. You'll be asking them a lot of questions, and if your parents are over eighty-five (part of the "frail elderly"), one or both of them may have little left of their short-term memory. Statistically one in two Americans have some form of dementia at this age. All this may generate much confusion, and your parents may just shut down.

None of us has limitless resources. Your patience and good humor will last longer if you lower your expectations of what you can get accomplished each time you're with them. You must stay focused. It helps for you to come there with your agenda ready, but even so, they may not be in the mood. It's likely you'll have a great deal to unearth at your parents' home, and perhaps, like me, a job, a family, and other responsibilities to return to. But you will want to be thorough and not discover later on that you forgot to look at the important boxes in the garage. The questions you don't get answered may rise again to haunt you another day.

Asking your parents the most personal and prying of questions takes courage. You may be way outside your comfort zone. You may be way outside their comfort zone too. You will need to ask and sometimes even pursue your parents for information they may not remember or want you to know. They may even become oppositional and refuse to grant you access to their secrets. Here's where you may find yourself face-to-face with the POParenting "role reversal," as you pursue with courage, patience, and determination the answers appropriate for a POParent to know.

You may be afraid they will get angry with you or feel offended. Maybe they will. Now is the time you can assure them with kindness that doing this is odd for you too. Instead of interrogating them about topics you've never talked about together, remind them (and yourself) that your concern is for their welfare and their future. You simply wish to help; you're not there to judge them. You might even ask them to be understanding with you. You can remind them that you are on a learning curve and you'll get more comfortable and confident as time goes by.

Remember, too, that it is you who can set—and should set—the right tone for these conversations. You are not cross-examining guilty prisoners; these are your parents.

Brace yourself for the fact that much of their paperwork may not be in shipshape condition. Perhaps your parents haven't been thinking very far ahead. Your questions can help them face up to important issues, think through, and then effectuate a better resolution of those—with you as a guide. Your parents may be feeling embarrassed to have you discover their unpaid insurance premiums, unopened bills, how much money they have, or the quantity of stored newspapers they're hoarding. You will want to be the calm and patient one, the understanding parent you always wanted to have when you were growing up. You'll want to keep your voice loud enough so they can hear your questions but not sound harsh or angry if you have to repeat yourself to be heard or comprehended.

If you're one of the fortunate POParents not facing the kind of drama or trauma that I did, benefiting from my story, you can have your initial conversations with your folks sufficiently early to understand what will be needed and do your research in a more relaxed manner. You can be better prepared than I was. You can take time to evaluate their home for its safety, help your parents draw up the most useful legal documents, meet with their doctors early on to prevent or slow the onset of certain geriatric conditions, and discover resources before your POP emergency or crisis arises.

5

DOING AND UNDOING PAPERWORK

Making Our Parents Safer and
Part of the Twenty-First Century

MY STORY

Despite having paid for my law school education and having frequently expressed confidence in me, my parents excluded me
when it came to drafting their wills and making their legal and
estate decisions. Now that my parents were finally including me in
these decisions and discussions, I needed to understand and perhaps offer my own input to what already existed. Maybe they
would wish to alter some things that would be more relevant to the
octogenarians they'd become and the world they found themselves in.

Hence, my first goal in reviewing their paperwork was to offer
my suggestions. My other goal was to ensure that going forward
we could all rely on my parents' documents, including with regard
to their wishes should another or more serious illness impact one
of them. Bottom line: while they were on my watch, I wanted my
parents to be and feel as safe as they could legally, emotionally,
spiritually, medically, and financially.

Given my legal background, I knew I'd feel more at ease after I took the time to fully examine their paperwork to see whether it was all in good order. I was coming to appreciate that as I became more serene and secure about each piece of the POP puzzle, my parents also became more at ease.

When I began the process, I had limited information. I knew things in the abstract, such as: my Dad held various rights and responsibilities from his music businesses that I'd need to learn about. I recalled hearing years before that they'd made a few small investments aside from their home, and I'd need to know if those were still active and what was involved. I remembered that in his early eighties Dad had proudly announced obtaining long-term care insurance for himself and Mom. "With this plan, you won't be burdened because our care will be assured." It was very important to my parents, as to many of their peers, not have to rely financially on their children, nor to obligate us in that way. I knew I'd need to check the details of their plan's premiums, benefits, waiting periods, and terms to see if his dream fit the insurance world's reality.

One day while I was hunting down information, I became so upset that I thought I might scream. It wasn't really that I wanted to scream—not at my parents, nor even at life. Rather, the tension I'd internalized burned in the muscles of my upper arms and I felt emotionally overwhelmed and claustrophobic in this storage cubicle, which was actually my mother's closet. A panicky feeling of not knowing what to do next, wanting to escape and feeling rooted in place, overcame me. I even heard myself silently revving up a host of unwanted emotions: "Ya know, Jane. Given your parents' pace, you might be here undoing and redoing rubber bands and forsaken files for months."

Some of the pressure came from the fact that these were not my therapy patients, with whom I could be the cool, competent professional. The stress I felt to do this POP task perfectly was so intense because it was my own Mom and Dad and because I knew I should be the calm and rational one, the parent, even in the midst of chaos.

And those endless boxes! What I found as I got inside Mom's boxes were decades and decades of memorabilia as well as financial, legal, and other extraordinarily detailed records. That woman, God love her, had saved not only every bank statement since their marriage but every letter I'd ever written her. She'd even saved the envelopes bearing their five-cent stamps and the new zip codes.

Jack made his own contribution to the collection of boxes I needed to examine. In addition to his stamp collection and random small coins he'd gathered, most of Dad's things consisted of the remnants of a background music library business he'd developed in his sixties. At that time, writing lyrics became less lucrative for a man his age, but he wanted to keep his hand in music and this business provided him a means. It also generated voluminous contracts, correspondence, tapes, CDs, and even vintage vinyl in foreign languages—Spanish, Bulgarian, and Swedish.

When I finally got inside the boxes that contained their personal legal papers, I was startled to learn that my parents' entire financial plan was based upon the man owning and controlling everything. Although Lillian had typed each piece of Dad's correspondence and every contract to precise perfection on an old Smith Corona typewriter—when a single error might require her retyping an entire page—Mom had no money. She had no credit, owned nothing and, despite having worked alongside Jack in all his business ventures, was basically not a "person" from a business perspective.

How could my fair-minded father have structured their assets that way? How could Mom or their lawyer have allowed it? The man I knew never denied Lillian's contribution to his life or business. Quite the contrary. He also wouldn't have set up their affairs with so little regard for Mom's well-being. In spite of my dismay, I decided our developing relationship would benefit if I responded more neutrally to things I was finding out. I had taught myself and then my patients to underreact rather than overreact at times with our younger family members. Certainly, I could learn to do that with these oldsters as well.

Helping my folks move into the twenty-first century was also part of my POP challenge, and it seemed likely I'd be more "persuasive" in getting them on board with POP if I underreacted more often. I could underreact by assuming anything I found that reflected Dad's sole ownership was set up in an old-school way by a man who took pride in providing for his wife. I could underreact when I reminded myself that Jack had acted out of a traditional point of view. There wasn't anything mean-spirited in his intentions. As I underreacted more, tempering my expression of emotions, I saw myself becoming more successful in obtaining their consent to the changes that were needed.

Helping myself move into the POParent I wished to become was not quite so easy. On the previous day, as I'd stood amid their things, I'd felt like an alien suspended above Mom's closet, looking down on this scene and asking myself: "What are you doing here, Jane, inside this closet in this bedroom sorting through years of these people's papers, photos, stamp collections, shoe boxes, music, and books?" Could that bizarre "dislocation" have come from a desire to avoid my feelings? My parents were not "these people." They were *the* two people I'd known the longest, the ones who'd conceived me, raised me as best they could, and shepherded me through my early life. But thinking about them as "these people" allowed me to distance myself from them and my feelings, feelings I sought to protect myself from having.

Gazing over the boxes, I identified those unwanted thoughts and emotions: exhaustion, sadness, nostalgia, and even anticipatory grief about their deaths. In that moment, I felt as if parenting my parents was part of an inevitable march toward their leaving me. Leaving *me*. Even Mom's not being recognizable on that first December night could be seen as part of *my* loss: the Mom I'd known seemed to be departing from my life.

My mind next jumped further into the scary future, to when I would be the old woman. What would my life accumulations look like to those sorting and reviewing my things? And who would be there to do this for me then?

"Whoa!" I told myself, noting I was not in the present. That type of thinking stripped away my positive energy and focus and therefore was actually dangerous behavior. I breathed a few times, deeply in and out. Then I tried another technique that I taught in my office: helpful self-talk. "Hey, you're not an old woman. Your parents are not dying. You're not operating in real time. Come on back." Breathing deeply into these present-centered cues helped ground me to where I was standing in the here and now, needing to function.

It was helpful to recognize my own mental patterns of succumbing to emotions of loss and abandonment, obsessively asking unanswerable questions. When I got lost in them, I was unable to mindfully attend to either my tasks or my parents. Once I'd uncovered these sometimes hard-to-identify patterns, I could intervene to bring me back to the present, since being "absent" is never a good formula for POParenting—or any other kind of parenting.

I was buoyed having witnessed the power that I had to fight my destructive and enervating thoughts. That evening, I continued to work on finding the desired energy and confidence needed to be the POParent I desired to become. I used more helpful "self-talk," as we psychotherapists call this skill, to show me how to undermine my distracted thinking.

Conversing inwardly again, I reminded myself: "You have what it takes to be the grown-up here. Surely you can tolerate Dad's having not made Mom a financial equal, and you can live with her annoying rubber band obsession. You can be the calm one and give your parents a sense of well-being. Reviewing legal and financial issues, sorting out health matters, and listening to people's spiritual concerns—these are all things you're particularly qualified to do. You've performed similar tasks successfully countless times, and now it's time to do it for your own loved ones. Calm down, Jane, you know what you're doing. You're fine."

These thoughts did ground me, and as I got more centered, I realized that not only had I been obsessively repeating unanswerable queries but also that I'd been asking all the wrong questions. I'd been dwelling on the "why me" questions and the "am I adequate" fears. These only convinced me to feel like a victim and not up for the job—things that weren't so. I was *not* a victim here: quite the opposite! I had fully chosen to help Lillian and Jack. Asking myself the wrong questions, like "am I enough?" and "why me?" wasn't helpful to anyone.

In contrast, posing the "right questions" would help me create much-needed empowering and solution-oriented responses. Those more constructive self-inquiries would involve asking my-self questions about HOW to proceed. "How can I sort through what I need from these boxes and still return to L.A. fairly soon?" "How can I find someone to help me with this?" "How could I make this more fun? Would turning on some music help us all have a better time?" "Would it work better to look for things myself and not bother Mom and Dad?"

Working as a therapist, I'd consistently found asking "how" questions to be a great way to generate action-oriented thoughts. By interrupting the "why me" questions and inserting the far more useful "how" questions, I was not only relieved of unhelpful men-tal meanderings but also able to focus on getting specific results. By asking myself "how" I could best complete the daunting POP tasks before me, I was actively commanding my mind to find good solutions. It was actually easier to get my job done.

After working with myself on these reorientations of my think-ing that day and later at the hotel, a more mature and confident version of me arrived at my parents' door the following day, a "wiser POParent." I was able to keep my attention mindfully poised on each step of what I was doing. Instead of judging my parents for having so much stuff or myself for not being a more patient POParent, I quieted those voices and just did my job. Very patiently I examined the next box in front of me, rather than losing myself in the overwhelming responsibility of "endless" boxes and work.

During the days that followed, I found more ways to motivate myself to clear out my stale, unwanted thoughts. I could clear my head quickly by going outside to take a brief and conscious walk as a personal time-out. Literally putting myself into a different space and moving my body offered a simple, nontoxic solution. Something else I tried in order to put me into another time and space was inviting my mind to clear itself of the thought of their apartment as it was today with its endless boxes, anxious parents, and disarray. In its place I brought in another scene from years ago, a specific and happy memory of what it had been like to live in Manhattan with my parents when I'd been young. I saw that I had many happy memories to choose from, and after allowing myself some time to savor a good memory, I could return to my tasks in their apartment refreshed and surprisingly efficient.

Unfortunately, even after I'd found the time to review my parents' paperwork and offered them some suggestions that we incorporated, I was not peaceful. I suffered from a condition I would see so often among POParents that I even gave it a name: "Insufficient Information Syndrome," or IIS. Although no one in business or law would advise making important decisions without hard data, there was no hard data on many crucial things. Instead I suffered from IIS, as I had no idea, of course, how long my parents would live or how their needs might expand. How long would any funds my parents had set aside for their late-in-life care last? How fast and often would the escalating cost of everything geriatric rise?

I closed my eyes, took a breath, and asked myself the question I'd often heard Oprah ask others. "What do you know for sure?" I did know this: I was "in" for the long haul. I had whatever resources I could locate, and it was my responsibility to figure out how to use those for my parents' well-being. I knew for sure that I'd keep them safe as best I could. I'd just have to find a way to live with my IIS and make the best decisions I could with whatever data I possessed.

These early POP days were a wealth of training opportunities for me, demonstrating clearly that what I'd been telling others was right for me, too. I saw that when I returned on future visits, I'd need to come prepared—calm, purposeful, and focused—since showing up like that allowed my parents to be clearer and even better able to help. I was appreciating that I could only accomplish a limited number of tasks during any one visit. If I tried to do too much, tempers would flare and the quality of our time together would suffer. People my parents' age moved and thought at a slower pace, and it was I, not they, who would need to do the adjusting.

It became clear that I would benefit from further practicing "emotional neutrality," underreacting, employing positive self-talk and that I could use some additional work on my patience. I'd found it hard to keep serene, and I didn't like how little emotional stamina I'd had recently. I would need to get help from my friends and family, the people who ordinarily let me vent, to talk through things without censoring. Hopefully doing all that would allow me to reemerge stronger.

Eventually we redid the paperwork, where needed. The Wolfs were now logging into the twenty-first century. Mom became a full partner in the family funds and developed a credit status at age eighty-five. I gained access to their accounts and, should they become unable, to making their medical decisions. I assured my parents that all their new documents were properly executed and stored and we all breathed another sigh of relief. This POP stage had been successfully completed.

Finally able to look up from the boxes, I gazed toward the ceiling in their bedroom and saw anew the state of their apartment. My Mom had refused permission for workers to come in to repaint and, over time, the discolored Sheetrock on the ceiling had become visible. That would have to wait for another visit.

YOUR STORY

You too will want to find, read, consider, and then discuss with family members what your parents have set in place, legally, financially and beyond. Depending on their circumstances, you may wish to include your parents in that process. Thereafter, you'll want to examine any reasonable alternatives to see if there are more current, less expensive, or other better ways to modify your parents' existing situations. You will want to do this sooner rather than later, since making and executing these decisions often takes time, an unknown here, and your parents may have a limited window to possess the mental competency necessary to change their documents.[1]

First, you'll need to find out all about your parents' finances. What are their assets and where are they located? Just because your father says he has an interest in an oil well in Texas or one of those certificates of ownership in Jack Daniels' land doesn't mean its value is what he's thinking. Do you know if your parents' assets are insured? If so, by what company and under what conditions? That information may also help you evaluate its worth. What are your parents' premiums, deductibles, and benefits for all their insurance? Do your parents have debt or mortgage obligations? Do they have a reverse mortgage, and is that working for them? Who are they paying, for what, and from what source? We all hear about older citizens getting ripped off. Has that happened to your parents? Are their bills being paid on time? How do you know that? Do they have debt, and if so, how is it being managed? Is it at a good rate? You will need to see their paperwork for yourself and attend to what is necessary.

Your parents may have become more forgetful, gotten ill, or just had trouble keeping track of their mail and so much more. As a result of their forgetfulness, for example, they may not be paying money they owe to some federal agency or their nondeductible portion of a hospital bill. If so, you'll need to understand which of your parents' bills must be paid immediately and what may be renegotiated by you later. You will want to ensure that no bills get lost lying around at your parents' home somewhere. Your aging parents' priorities may sometimes surprise you: to them, being late for dinner may be unthinkable but being late on a car insurance premium may be "no big deal."

If you can't get reliable answers from your parents about their existing monthly payments, you'll want to create a theoretical list of their likely obligations. For example, if your parents own their home, they may owe on a mortgage or two, an equity line, or a reverse mortgage. You will then need to go find such documents and seek out specific answers. If your parents are still driving, they may owe payments on an auto lease or a loan. A car registration or a smog check may be coming due soon. Once you've gotten a handle on their bills, it would be helpful to put reminder cues in place on a central calendar you create for recurring events so that whoever starts to pay their bills can do so in a timely manner.

If your review of their current situation suggests your folks are unable to continue managing their finances without ongoing help, you may need to take over some or all of it. You also may wish to consult an attorney and see about filing a petition in court seeking a conservatorship of their money or whatever their state requires for you to manage their finances, especially if you're concerned about your parents' signing checks or making poor financial choices. A power of attorney may be sufficient but you will want to have certainty to best protect yourself, your parents, and their estate.

Having "the Conversation" with your parents about your taking on more control of their money or other aspects of their life usually has many levels of complexity to it. Again, harkening back to parenting children, you have a moral obligation, should you choose to accept it, to protect your parents financially. That may mean that your being cosignees on their bank accounts is necessary at this time of your POPcycle. You will also want to protect them from scams, missed payments, or other unattractive consequences. Under more unfortunate circumstances, you may even need to protect your parents from a sibling who's living under their roof and "conning" them out of their Social Security moneys.

After having reviewed your parents' obligations, resources, and foreseeable needs, perhaps you will suggest that they obtain a personal loan or a reverse mortgage on their home. A low interest rate may present an attractive solution to finding the funds you need to hire caregiving assistance. Perhaps you'll advise your parents to make some short-term investments to extend the life of their savings. You will want to keep current regarding taxes, Social Security, and Medicare. There are many resources available to

help you including, of course, the POP website, http://www.
ParentingOurParents.org .

It's wise to spend some funds in the beginning of your POPcycle to have experienced professionals guide you and your family—
evaluating what's in place, legally and financially, and deciding
what might be better. Perhaps someone on your TEAM POP already has these skills, but if not, find qualified people licensed in
the state where your parents are planning to live out their days.
There may even be legal or financial professionals providing free
advice for the indigent elderly in their state; your parents may or
may not qualify for these services. In making financially prudent
choices, it's often wise to expend some money now to ensure future savings will exist and to avoid stressful worrying. Even if you
and/or your parents have concerns about the expense, you may
find it useful and comforting to consult with seasoned professionals.

Over the course of your POPcycle, you will likely find yourself
hiring, firing, and supervising lawyers, doctors, accountants, geriatric care managers (GCMs), and others. They may have far more
education and certainly will have far more experience in their
areas of expertise than you do. Supervision of these professionals
in the form of oversight and follow-up is part of POParenting and
it is the job of the whole TEAM POP. The best-qualified or most
local TEAM POP member is often the one to be assigned such
overseeing. I urge you as POParents to not become intimidated by
professionals who are helping your family. Speak up! Ask a lot of
questions! Better safe asking too many questions than sorry asking
too few. It's your job to ensure that your parents are getting the
best service possible, so don't let your old fearfulness stand in the
way of good POParenting.

Knowing that you've become involved, that their paperwork
has been updated, that they're not alone dealing with their hospital bills or balancing their bank books *will* relieve your loved ones'
stress. That can literally extend the number and the quality of your
parents' days and nights on the planet.

6

FACING DOWN THE LIFE-AND-DEATH MISSION OF POP—THEIRS AND YOURS

MY STORY

I was at home one afternoon doing nothing in particular when an unrelenting voice in my head kept repeating: "Call Dad NOW!" Ordinarily when I thought about him, I'd smile and remind myself to call. "Gee, it'd be nice to speak to Dad. I must remember to phone him later, when I get the chance." But this time something about it seemed urgent.

I obeyed.

Florence, our caregiver, picked up the phone and formally announced: "Wolf residence."

"Hi, Florence. I'm looking for my Dad. Is he okay? Will you go tell him I'm calling, please?" I sounded cool, but my heart was beating loudly in my chest. I was focused and uninterested in chatting with Florence, as I ordinarily would have done to gain her view on the current situation with my folks. Now I just wanted to feel the relief of hearing my dear daddy's voice. I had a very cold feeling crawling up my back and chest.

Florence got back on the line to tell me she couldn't find him.

Now my heart was jumping out of my chest. "*No!* Go find him!" Florence disappeared again. It was not a very big place, so he couldn't be lost! They only had a two-bedroom apartment! What the . . . !

Florence returned breathless. It turned out that Dad had quietly slipped into my former bedroom, aka his music business office, and locked himself inside. Responding to my demands, Florence burst in on him and found that he had placed a plastic bag over his sad bald head. He'd been trying to end his life!

I grasped the enormous importance of my being alert to my own internal voice and willingness to respond by calling. What if I had not been alert to my internal voice? What if I had dismissed that relentless urging? What if I had not phoned? What if Florence had not been there?

I am so grateful that I heeded my nagging voice on that otherwise "do-nothing" afternoon. Somehow, I'd felt it, that instinctive signal parents describe getting when their kids are in danger. Perhaps my close POP attachment to Dad had in a similar way alerted me that something was very wrong, even thousands of miles away.

I was already having serious doubts about the long-distance POP I was trying to do. Maybe it wasn't my finest idea. In fact, the afternoon's events seemed not only a blessing in having saved Jack but perhaps also a wake-up call: I would need to be watching more carefully than before, more than I could even imagine. And since my parents didn't want to leave New York, my greater oversight would have to come from a distance.

Dad's behavior had truly shaken me up. I'd been totally unprepared for him to become so beaten down by life's stressors that he would contemplate suicide as his last life statement. He'd been "the rock" for everyone else since his childhood, helping his kid brothers, buying up my uncle's cleaning business. "Dependable Jack," they'd called him. "Mr. Moderation," as Jack sometimes called himself, wasn't the kind of guy to take his own life. But somehow over the prior several months, when I'd expected Jack and Lillian to settle into their more protected life, my ever-stable father had been acting in dangerously uncharacteristic ways.

Even with the abiding humility he cultivated, Jack had always seemed bigger than life to me. Maybe most girls feel that way about their daddies. Looking back at the time, I remembered how his being ever curious about everyone and everything had meant I couldn't pull my dates away from talking with him. When had he stopped being curious? He had always seemed so comfortable being the strong, invincible one. Had he tired of the role? Only once in my whole life had I ever seen him cry. Dad had become totally frustrated over something rather small, but it had gotten to him and he just sat and wept. It was eerie to watch as a child, but the incident also humanized him for me. I'd never seen a serious break in him before. Nor had I foreseen that of my two parents it would be Dad whom I would need to rescue from a suicide attempt.

I was shocked and profoundly saddened that he'd felt so desperate that he wanted to end his life. Of course, I jumped on the next plane to New York. I had no idea what I would do when I got there or what I'd actually say to him. I'd figure those things out in the moment. Now I just wanted to hold his hand, take him on a walk in Central Park, and offer him the peacefulness he used to give me when I needed rescuing as a child.

Maybe Dad would share his burdens or disappointments with me. I also felt badly for not having been more aware. I'd not seen his unhappiness, and he'd never confided it to me. I was shocked that he'd think suicide could be a solution. I wondered if he'd been thinking at all or just reacting. Maybe he was just feeling forlorn and overwhelmed. I feared that even when I was by his side, Dad—like so many men of his generation—wouldn't communicate very much about his emotions. I also wondered how much, if at all, I could help him.

By the time I got into Manhattan from the airport, Dad had been calmed down from his suicide attempt. He was grateful to have me there and told me he appreciated my answering his "call for help." I'd naively hoped that some of the fatigue, withdrawal from life, and absence of joy I'd seen at Christmastime would clear up after his daughter and the caregivers improved his life. However, this depression had not abated much at all.

None of it had truly lightened the internal burdens Jack had placed on himself, it seemed to me now. Trying unsuccessfully to be his wife's caregiver, Dad had to face that his wife and life partner had been diagnosed with Alzheimer's and there was little he could do about that but watch the decline and love her. This news had taken its toll on the resilient man he had always been.

Depression is often hard to detect for family members even if you're living nearby, and it's even harder from a distance. As I looked back, there had been clues that Dad's stress and life changes could turn into a major depressive episode. And statistically, there is a remarkably high rate of suicides (and attempts) among men in their eighties. But even I, the thorough professional therapist, had wanted to believe things were getting better and had not been looking for signs of depression in my father, my strong parent. And of course, I wasn't there to observe him. But even had I been physically closer, suicide attempts are complicated phenomena and not necessarily predictable, despite someone's depressed mood.

At this point in life, Dad was entering his late eighties and still working at his background music publishing business. It was very detail-oriented work, involving foreign rights and domestic contracts. My folks had been a team in that business from the beginning. As Mom's cognitive decline became more apparent, she was less able to keep up her end of the tasks. I could see how her condition might have distressed and challenged Dad, demanding additional unknown skills from him at an age when he was finding it harder to learn new things. A man half his age would have had problems carrying on their projects (without his partner) and persevering despite grieving.

When I began POP, so much of my attention had been focused on Mom and the impact of her dementia on her activities of daily living, her moods, and her functioning. Now I'd been forced to pull the camera lens farther back on the scene and see the effects of Mom's conditions on our larger family dynamics. Jack too had aged over the past visits. Caring for his ailing, aging beloved wife had stressed him and made him more vulnerable, first to pneumonia and later to depression. Despite Florence's continuing attention, it was mostly my father upon whom my mother relied for real support, and her long-term cognitive illness also seemed to be impacting his emotions.

It couldn't have been easy for him. I tried to get my father to talk with me as we walked through Central Park. It was not his practice to "burden" his child. But after I'd so quickly returned to be with him in New York, Dad began to talk more, although in a limited way, acknowledging feelings of confusion, loss, resentment, and even shame. I listened, offered an occasional interjection, and listened more. I held his hand, kissed his bald head, and reminded him of my steadfast love and appreciation. There was only so much I could do for him, even as I wanted to do more.

During my mother's long cognitive decline, Dad had needed to become her primary caregiver and, as a result, he had needed to give up a central part of their marital arrangement: their working partnership. Dad was beginning to learn that medication could slow Mom's dementia for a while, but that as time went by, she would become less and less his wife. Florence's calming demeanor was very helpful for both of them around their house. Her quiet consistency and the predictable patterns she created worked well for both my folks, in spite of their very different personalities and needs.

On this visit, more clearly than ever, I'd come to see that, since I couldn't rely on my parents to be accurate reporters of their own conditions, and since as a POParent I had a pressing need to know, it was my job to develop more reliable and regular procedures to oversee them at a distance. Florence and I created a protocol in which I'd be quickly alerted to any observable changes in my parents' behaviors or health. She prepared written reports weekly. I advised their building's superintendent to have the staff on the lookout for anything "unusual" with my parents, especially on the weekends when they were "home alone." I was battening down the hatches around the boat carrying my fragile folks.

Even though I held onto the hope that Dad would feel like his former self after his suicidal attempt, he clearly needed more help.

I checked into some psychiatric referrals for him and set up an appointment a few days later. Then I went home. Flying back to New York to be with him had only provided a temporary fix, it seemed. I returned to California, enjoyed a good night's sleep in my own bed, and then heard the phone ring the next morning, very early. It was Dad.

"If you don't come back, I'm going to kill myself."

What would I do now? What would the experts advise? But I was supposed to be the expert! This is why doctors don't treat their own families, I reminded myself. I was hardly objective.

Nonetheless, I looked to see how I, the geriatric expert as well as the daughter who adored him, could best help. I recognized that I must take his threats seriously, especially after his recent episode, but somehow this didn't feel like the time before. This time it felt like what parents get when their child needs more of their attention. Was Dad truly suicidal or was he making some desperate attempt to test me? If he were truly suicidal again, the day after I returned home, then I would need to have Florence get him to an institution. If, on the other hand, he just needed more of my attention, then I was in parent-child territory, and I had some good ideas of what to do next.

I went with my gut and my new role-reversing mantra: "You're their parent now!" It didn't really feel like Dad wanted to kill himself, despite his words. It really sounded like he wanted me around more. I asked myself how could I best respond to him lovingly but also with appropriate limits, like a practiced POParent. I wanted him to know I was there for him but that I couldn't be bounced back and forth across country. I couldn't afford to get this wrong.

Very carefully, I decided to try employing with my beloved Dad some of the coaching techniques I'd already developed for patients who were POParenting. Soon thereafter, I would flesh out these techniques to create the curriculum for the POP Family Coaching program. Today, there are certified POP Family Coaches helping families—like yours—nationwide. As a result, I was able to "multiply myself" by sharing my successful POP coaching tools with many more families so their POPcycles could be both more workable and more loving. We continue to expand the numbers of certified POP coaches, many of whom have themselves been POParents; and, all of whom aim to do their part to undermine the damage of the silver tsunami we've already begun experiencing.

The first technique I tried with Jack was the "test question": "What age is your parent behaving as, right now?" I found that even asking that question calms POParents down by allowing them to put a little distance in place. Interestingly, by taking a moment to consider your aging parents' "childish" ways, and perhaps also recalling similar ways your kids acted, you can find an actual number your parent is behaving as: a very powerful tool, I had observed many times before, in my office.

Now, I thought to ask myself: "What age is Jack now?" And somehow, quite naturally, my mind answered. I instantly knew the age that seemed closest to how Jack was acting. It was about eight. If you've ever seen an eight-year-old boy act somewhat irrationally, desperate for his mother's attention, that was pretty similar to what Dad was evoking in that moment. How does a parent treat an eight-year-old boy who's feeling needy?

Over time, I'd also seen how helpful it was for me and lots of POParents to use the technique of underreacting. I applied that technique as well. Then, I took the deepest cleansing breath I could muster and made myself sound as kind and normal as I could: "Do you think you could wait all the way until next weekend, Dad, for me to come back and for us to spend some time together? I've just returned home and that means I just can't turn around and return to New York without at least seeing my office and some of my patients. I know the weekend may seem like a long time, but I promise that if you won't be too sad until then, I will come back this weekend. Can you work with me on that?"

I set a boundary but was still holding my breath to hear his response. I had no idea if my approach would work or if he would hang up and try to hurt himself. I hoped he would give in to the reasonableness of my request and get that I'd heard his neediness and would soon be back.

"Okay. I'll wait. And Jane, thank you."

As it turned out, Dad's depression was not remedied. Over a period of months, he would try to kill himself on three separate occasions—once by plastic bag and then twice more by leaning out the window of the fourteenth-floor duplex apartment he'd fought so hard to get into. The last attempt he almost jumped, knowing I was in a cab across town on my way to see him. But he didn't jump, thank God!

Over those months, I'd unearthed various specialists for Dad to meet with in addition to his prescribing psychiatrist. He saw psychologists, clinical social workers, and religious men. He took biofeedback treatments, psychiatric medications, and herbal supplements to prevent future harm, alleviate existing symptoms, and function better. But, poor man, he still seemed to be crying out for additional help.

One way I hoped to provide him help was to relieve him of the burden associated with his music publishing business. Perhaps if given the chance, I could sell off the valuable assets he'd written and published but now lacked the energy to exploit commercially. After having appropriately compensated Dad for his copyrights, perhaps the new, younger publisher would also want to use Jack's considerable veteran expertise to further advise him. With fewer responsibilities, the pride associated with unexpected funds in the bank, and the respect that came with being a consultant, Jack might experience a reason to live, an RTL.

It took me a long time to accomplish, but eventually I was able to sell Dad's published work to people who continued to share it with the listening public. His joy in that transaction and all the accompanying benefits of it lit up my world.

Another way I hoped to relieve some of Dad's emotional burdens, and Mom's too, was through the mentoring and support I got from colleagues. Throughout my POP journey, I was blessed to have Dr. Michael L. McGrail as my geriatric guru. A devoted friend and my office partner, Michael was a highly gifted psychiatrist with an amazingly kind heart and a devilish sense of humor, who was beloved by his patients and students. Having him by my side while parenting my parents was a gift, as Michael always provided me both the information I needed for POP and the wisdom to interpret the data accurately. I would call him day or night from the emergency rooms of hospitals—sometimes desperate and always grateful for his sound advice.

After so many attempts to treat Dad weren't helping, Michael convinced me that Dad's form of depression would best be halted by carefully administered electroshock treatments (EST). No longer the frightening experience portrayed in 1950s movies, EST had become an acceptable last-ditch way to permanently relieve intense psychological pain. When Dad tried suicide a third time, I agreed to the treatment. I can recall few sadder moments in my whole life than leaving my daddy to be prepped for these shock treatments.

Tied down to a "geri-chair"—one of those hospital high chairs where old people look like young children waiting for lunch— Jack's eyes were deeply sunken and radiated terror. I wanted so badly to comfort him, to make it all better for the man who'd been there to comfort me and my "boo-boos" in his day. I let Dad know that he would feel better again soon and would function more like himself after the treatments. I suggested he talk frankly with the nice young woman who was the social worker, confiding that she shared my training and might become one of his best allies on the road to recovery. He said he would try.

With a very heavy heart, I left him sitting in that high chair and headed back to their apartment. There I bid farewell to Mom who was a bit confused with all the psychiatric attention now focused on Jack. I checked in again with Florence and told her to be on the lookout for Mom's need for some special attention. Then I went down to the building superintendent and instructed him to install bars on the windows of my parents' elegant apartment. That would assure that neither parent could use their fourteenth-floor windows as an exit point from this world. Then I boarded another plane, thankful to escape back to my home.

How much any of those treatments or professionals helped my father is frankly hard to assess and may not matter. I was grateful for anything that brought him some respite. Participating with these methodologies provided Jack a variety of tools to manage his stress and the more "single" life he would increasingly live as Mom retreated into her dementia. Jack never suffered a recurrence of his symptoms, to my great relief.

YOUR STORY

Hopefully, you will never have to be on a call like mine rescuing a potentially suicidal parent or loved one. But it is possible that you will as a part of doing POP. If it does happen to you, hopefully reading this information will alert you to handling it more effectively.

If you or your parent are having a personal crisis and need help right now, call this toll-free number: 1-800-273-TALK (8255). Your call goes directly to the National Suicide Prevention Hotline. All calls to this line are always confidential. Even if it seems totally unlikely, you should keep the number handy for future use.

POP, in reality, is a life-and-death mission with the end point your parents' departure from the planet. There will be times when, for everyone's sake, you may wish the end to come sooner rather than later. Seeing people you love in any kind of pain—physical, spiritual, or emotional—is hard, and sometimes you may want the suffering to end. If you have had such thoughts, do not feel bad. I repeat: *do not feel bad*. They are just thoughts. Thoughts are real and they are measurable, but they are not actions. Research teams have estimated that a person has as many as ninety thousand thoughts each day. And we all have thoughts from time to time that don't represent our finest hour. So, don't start punishing yourself for your thoughts.

If you are doing the primary family caregiving, like my Dad felt he was, there's a lot of information and many resources available about taking care of *you*! Family caregiving may often result in depression or some other health issue to the caregiver who rarely pays sufficient attention to him/herself. This is not an exaggeration. Like my Dad, one of your parents may already have joined the more than sixty-five million Americans (more than three in ten households) who provide unpaid care to an elderly or disabled adult family member.[1] These family caregivers provide an estimated 80 percent of the long-term care in the United States.

It is not at all uncommon for live-in family caregivers to develop serious health problems. Research has shown family caregivers are more likely than non-caregiving family members to:

- display symptoms of depression or anxiety
- have a long-term medical problem
- show higher levels of stress hormones
- spend more days sick with an infectious disease
- have a weaker immune response to flu vaccines
- heal wounds slower
- suffer from obesity
- show a higher risk of mental decline, including problems with memory and concentration (the precise areas one doing POP would most want most to have)

A few years ago I tried unsuccessfully to set up a support group for people doing POP. Prospective members told me they definitely wanted to feel better, could absolutely use support from fellow caregivers, and knew they *should* give some loving attention to themselves. But they were unwilling to commit to regularly attending a group whose focus would be on their own well-being and not their parents. Just as you and I, when we were young parents, set our "default" to attend to our baby first, when parenting aging parents, many family caregivers similarly take care of parents first, bathing, feeding, and attending to ourselves much later, if ever.

Promise yourself that you won't fall into this pattern of self-neglect. Find ways to set some boundaries or space between you and the loved ones you take care of. Schedule at least some activities that are focused on you alone. Make some time every day to attend to you, even if it's only a quiet cup of tea as you listen to a favorite piece of music. You will recall that on airplane flights, when instructing about emergency oxygen masks, they always remind parents: put your own on first. Similarly, with family caregiving: if you don't take care of you, you may not be ready when it's time to help your parents!

If you're a spouse to a senior or an older adult child of one, remember that your poor self-care may eventually make you more at risk than the person you're attending! Yes, some caregivers will die before their charges. And what good will you be to your loved ones—and what sort of model—if you become ill or disabled and then need a caregiver of your own?

If your senior parents are still living with a partner, the fact that people age at very different rates may have an effect on them as a couple as well as individuals. People decline at different rates, partly because of genetics and partly because of different lifestyles and mental attitudes. Even if your mother and father have the same number of years on the planet, as mine did, they may now be functioning at and feeling themselves to be very different "ages." I see many situations where the husband persists in his provider role by taking care of his same-age or even younger wife. Contrary to many of our stereotypes, one in every three American family caregivers is male.[2]

Your parents may conspire, consciously or less so, as mine did in the beginning, to keep their limitations hidden from you, the outsider. That may take the form of covering up what's forgotten and then compensating by trying to fill in the blanks when they can't recall details. For example, your dad may claim he phoned you yesterday as promised, even supplying details, when he doesn't really remember. Partners will often camouflage each other's disabilities, making your detection of conditions like depression harder. This is a version of how your teenage children may have acted, although for very different reasons. Perhaps back then you honed your "parental detectors" and can now utilize them for POP. Your aging parents may be falsely reasoning that they can hold on to their autonomy, their home, and their lifestyle if they don't let any outsiders know about "weak links in their chain." But as we've seen, that is rarely, if ever, in their best interest.

Depression among the elderly is a very serious matter. It is widely associated with suicide. Older Americans are disproportionately likely to die by their own hand. White non-Hispanic men over seventy-five pose an unusually high risk for self-destruction.[3] This phenomenon is under-recognized and undertreated. Disturbingly, some health professionals and even some seniors themselves mistakenly believe that persistent depression is a normal way to live because of the serious illnesses and financial hardships that often accompany aging in our society. Many older adults who die by suicide visited a physician within a month before death, yet the signs of depression apparently went unheard. As a result, it's even more pressing for those doing POP to be alert to our parents' wake-up call.

This underscores the urgency of improving your ability to detect your beloved elderly parents' mood disorders. One of your goals in being a proficient POParent is to train yourself to use your "observing eye" in service of your aging loved ones. As you become attuned to the symptoms of geriatric depression, perhaps you can help avert a family crisis. Take the time now to review your parents' reactions—over the past several weeks. Note if your parents have had any changes in

appetite
weight
energy
concentration
sleep
mood patterns

or feelings of:

hopelessness
helplessness
lack of pleasure in things usually pleasurable (anhedonia)

Elderly people with severe depressive bouts are still over-whelmingly in the minority. If a number of these symptoms persist for two weeks or longer or they get worse over the weeks, your parents may be abnormally depressed. It is always worth checking out your concerns with their doctors since depressive disorder is *not* a normal part of the aging process. You will likely want to reevaluate any geriatric professional who tells you it is.

While everyone experiences sadness, grief, feelings of loss, and the occasional blue mood, persistent depression is different, and it is not normal. And although your parents may be very sad if and when their partners and long-standing friends die, generally speaking, people often feel more secure and content as they mature.

Those who lived into their eighties and nineties reported that their emotional happiness increased as they aged and, despite the high valuation we place on youthfulness, older Americans report being happier with their lives than younger people. A sample of twenty-eight thousand people interviewed from 1972 to 2004 revealed that the happiest sector of Americans is the oldest.[4] As they aged, older adults rated their life satisfaction much higher, with happiness ratings rising gradually and steadily from age fifty through the decade of the nineties. Researchers are calling this process the "U-curve" of happiness.[5]

A big part of POP involves your becoming watchful of your parents in a different way than you've ever been before. That may look like doing "watchful" things—examining their personal effects in ways that might have seemed like an imposition on their privacy when they were younger. You might look over their mail, check the contents of their cupboards and refrigerator, and inspect their medicine chests for information about undisclosed diseases and a better understanding of how much and which medicines they're taking. You may even wish to do some POP research by going online to read up on their prescription drugs and their side effects.

In your POParental role, your watchfulness may have to take on a subtler form as well. The next time you're around a caring parent with a very young child, watch the parent's eyes track the child's eyes and any change in the facial movements of the child. Similarly, as you watch a caring POParent mopping the brow of a dad who has forgotten his child's name, it is likely the POParent's eyes will also be tracking the father's eyes and any changes in his facial movements.

If you're going to do POP well, you may also need to supplement your own eyes and those of other family members with professional help, full-time or part-time. If so, your TEAM POP will need to address these questions now and again over time.

- What do our mom and dad require help doing now?
- How many days or hours/week do they need this help?
- When do we need to start to give them that help?
- How much will that cost and how are we/they going to afford it?
- If there isn't enough money, how else can we use our talent and resources to get them the help they require?

In order to oversee these various POP tasks and your parents' aides, you or someone in your family will soon be learning the ins and outs of these systems: Medicare, Medicaid, long-term care insurance, pensions from employment, geriatric dosages of medication, home health care workers, and more. We continue to provide updated resources, links, and blogs at the POP website (http://www.ParentingOurParents.org) so you can further explore what you will need for your folks. Online governmental resources also make it easier today for POParents to become conversant with terms like: eligibility guidelines, waiting periods, deductibles, and waivers. Your designated family member can apply for many programs online, including Social Security, and get much helpful information directly from the providers of the services.

You will want to be creating a TEAM POP contact list. Include as many people as you can on your list so that you have backup choices if needed. Make sure you get the cell phone numbers and email addresses for your parents' neighbors and close friends for the TEAM POP contact list you're developing. You may be pleasantly surprised at the kindness of neighbors who've lived across the hall from your parents for the last twenty years. They can sometimes add extraordinary eyes and ears where you can't be. Remember to keep your contact list updated with changes and to send the updated lists to everyone.

But no matter how many people you hire or who they are, *you* are still the one leading POP. As such, you need to remain watchful as things change, and they will change, of that you can be certain. If your parents have a good geriatric care manager (GCM), you may only need to be in regular and ongoing contact with one centralized source of information. Even if they have a GCM, you may be the type of POParent who wishes to have more direct and/or written protocols with your parents' caregivers and others to better monitor any changes. You may be watching as carefully as you can, but be aware that sometimes things change quickly in little ways that end up changing everything.

7

DISCOVERING OUR PARENTS MAY NEED TO LEAVE HOME

MY STORY

Jack and Lillian were home alone each weekend for several years. From Friday night after Florence left, having given them their dinners and medications, until Monday morning when she'd arrive in time to make them breakfast. My parents insisted that they would not accept a second caregiver after Florence left for the weekend. Even though I never supported this part of the POPlan—and it was the one real "hole"—I'd gone along to keep the peace.

Back at home in California, however, I was hardly peaceful. More accurately I walked around on eggshells every weekend during those years, worrying about them alone for all that time and waiting for my phone to ring. Although I wanted to, I knew I couldn't call every hour. A few times I actually chuckled, thinking this was my "payback"; as a teenager, I'd pooh-poohed my parents' demands to let them know I'd arrived somewhere safely. Now it was I who wanted them to call and check in. How ironic POP was turning out to be! But it made me laugh, and during POP laughter is almost always a real gift!

When I'd walked into the middle of the crisis that first Christmas, I had to respond immediately and with an infusion of massive help. In addition to the obvious need for a cleanup crew, the geriatric care manager (GCM) introduced me to a number of qualified professional caregivers who could be available for eight- or twelve-hour shifts. The GCM's suggestion had been to assign Dad a primary daytime person, Florence, and then use others to cover the remaining hours when she would be gone.

The GCM talked of "training" my parents to accept that they needed regular caregiving help even after they recovered from being sick. The GCM further argued we would need separate, additional full-time staffing for my mother after she returned from the hospital. How much would all this cost? Would each of my parents need a full-time individual attendant? And if so, why? I couldn't even figure out where all these people would stand in my parents' relatively small apartment?

On a more philosophical level, I also recognized that no matter how many caregivers I supplied my parents, I could never truly keep them safe forever. And what was "safe"? I saw that doing POP would involve my rediscovering the right balance any good parent aims to find: enough assistance and attention to provide safety and enough autonomy to promote their doing what they can for themselves.

Supporting as much self-reliance as was appropriate seemed to encourage my parents to do more for themselves. It also supplied a subtle but positive message that they still had much living left to do. This approach appropriately challenged my parents and seemed to be as helpful in POParenting as it had been in parenting my stepchildren when they were young. But it did require me to stay continually alert in order to achieve that right balance.

I would also need to discover how much caregiving assistance was right for them. Even before the thorough housecleaning was accomplished, I could see that my parents would require ongoing assistance. At the least, they'd need someone to keep their apartment clean and help them with their laundry, marketing, and meals. I intuitively sensed that too much help might be worse for my parents than not having enough, but I knew I didn't want them to be at either end of that continuum.

Upon Mom's return from the hospital, the GCM again expressed strongly her view that Lillian needed her own set of caregivers and needed them 24/7. Frankly I was concerned. Having that much help in my folks' home felt wrong for a series of reasons. My immediate reaction was that it felt like far too many eyes on my folks and they would hate that. They lived in a two-bedroom apartment with a modest amount of space. They'd feel overly watched with two caregivers there all day and every night, I suspected.

But I deferred to the GCM's superior experience. For once, I didn't listen to me. My private parents never liked much "oversight," and as a few days went by, I could feel them bridling against the rapt attention of ever-present caregivers. Hell, for years Mom hadn't even let in the guys she knew from the building to plaster the damaged ceilings.

Noting their current medical conditions and ages, I easily saw they'd need more help as time went by, so from a financial perspective, as well as other perspectives, I needed to find a level of help that we could maintain. If I spent what they'd set aside for their future care too quickly, we'd encounter a problem in the long run. Since I couldn't estimate how long a future we needed to plan for, that always made for complicated monetary planning.

My parents were receiving Social Security and Medicare, the two entitlement programs all US seniors are eligible to receive. But because of those programs' limitations in terms of health and long-term home care benefits, they also had to supplement the benefits they received from the government with additional coverage from private insurance companies. One covered them for the infamous Medicare "donut hole" gap in medication coverage.[1]

Fortunately for everyone concerned, Dad had purchased a long-term care (LTC) insurance policy for himself and Mom before they got into their eighties. If they had purchased these policies when they were younger, their premiums would have been lower. Nonetheless, having their LTC benefits helped out a lot, and doing POP led me to sign up for my own LTC policy. As soon as I saw how it helped my parents and made other POP choices more affordable for our family, I became an advocate. When I applied for my LTC policy, I was still young and took care to get the right policy for my predictable needs.

One wrinkle was that their LTC policy had a waiting period of ninety days after their claims were filed and their eligibility verified. During that waiting period, no benefits kicked in and my family had to pay out-of-pocket for all their help—domestic, GCM, caregiver, whatever wasn't covered by Medicare.

After my parents' LTC benefits commenced, we encountered another series of restrictions under their particular policy. First, their insurance company wouldn't pay for more than one caregiver. Second, Dad had mistakenly signed up for a policy that required him to continue making payments even after he and Mom were deemed sufficiently disabled to receive benefits. Third, Florence wasn't on the insurer's listing of accepted employees, known as their "registry." Only registry caregivers could receive payment under their LTC policy. And probably most troubling, the hourly fee paid to registry caregivers was less per hour than what we'd been paying Florence through the GCM.

Once I understood the contractual limitations of my parents' policy, I was left with several decisions. Should I continue paying for multiple caregivers with our funds or go along with the terms of their policy that afforded them only one caregiver? If I paid privately for two caregivers, clearly the funds we'd have for my parents' care would run out far more quickly. I decided to ask my parents' opinions.

Like many others who'd grown up in or lived through the Great Depression of 1929, they lived with the fear that their money would run out. They voted for one caregiver and that the person be Florence. Even before I'd asked, they'd complained that having people watch them sleep was an unnecessary waste. Mom particularly didn't like people "underfoot," as she called it and neither of them felt two people were necessary for their level of limitations. I found myself agreeing with their reasoning on this.

I'd hired the GCM to be my onsite eyes and ears, and we talked at length. The GCM was so unrelenting that I retain two caregivers 24/7 that she threatened to resign if I didn't follow her counsel. I felt really confused by the intensity of the GCM's reaction and was unnerved that she would talk of abandoning my parents over this decision.

That left me with a difficult quandary. I wanted sufficient attention for my parents but not excessive help that might actually weaken my parents. I didn't want to run out of money for their care—a frightening thought most POParents are plagued by—but also I didn't want to deprive them of what they needed because of funds. I appreciated the GCM's high standards for care if that was what she was arguing for. Maybe my folks and I were wrong. Perhaps they were so disabled that they needed that level of care? The last thing I wanted was to provide them insufficient caregiving attention.

And I felt particularly vulnerable: were there no GCM on the core team, I wasn't sure how well we'd do with our long-distance POPlan. Who would do the GCM's biweekly oversight visits? Since Mom and Dad seemed to be doing so well, I'd been feeling a bit more confident with my parents living so far away. Would I be putting their recoveries in jeopardy were I to cut back their caregiving to a single person, as was covered by their LTC insurance?

For my part, I didn't find it supportive to have our GCM threaten to "cut my parents loose" if we didn't choose her decisions. Where could I go for other reliable points of view? I talked with my geriatric mentor, psychiatrist Michael McGrail, who, by his experience with my parents' personalities and his professional insights, urged me to not overstaff my parents. I contacted my parents' long-standing doctors and even some of the people from their building to get an idea of what they were currently observing about my parents.

Finally, I listened to myself. I got rid of the double caregiving, let the GCM fire herself, and narrowed their staff down to one. That decision left me with my next set of challenges. Should I work with the insurance company to get Florence on their registry or start all over with one of the company's cheaper caregivers? If I were able to get Florence on to the insurer's registry, could I ask her to work for less money per hour than we'd originally agreed? And if I were able to get Florence on their registry in order to keep her working with my folks, could we afford to make up the difference between the insurer's hourly wages and the original hourly she was being paid through the GCM?

I saw how valuable Florence was and how well she worked with both my parents. They greatly encouraged me to find a way Florence could stay on with them. I got into "POP mode" and started negotiating with the LTC insurance company in order to get Florence onto their registry. When Florence agreed to do my parents' housecleaning and laundry, I was also able to cut back on the cleaning lady. By this point, we also weren't paying for the GCM. These changes left us in a budgetary position where I felt more comfortable supplementing Florence's registry hourly rate, which turned out to be a fine resolution for all concerned.

But like so many seemingly easy developments, little was easy when I was parenting my parents. Now I discovered there was one small wrinkle in this new "Florence only" POPlan. Lillian and Jack had drawn a line in the sand: "Nobody watches over us on the weekends. We like Florence, and that's okay, but we need our privacy too." While she was there from Mondays through Fridays, Florence was now my long-distance eyes and ears, but after she left, they were still *home alone* every weekend!

My parents were adults and they lived three thousand miles away. So, it appeared I had little choice, once they resisted my strong suggestions to have help for them on the weekends. What could I to do if they refused? It wasn't like I could demand they take a time out or ground them. But if they were hurt due to any lack of attention, I would feel terrible, and I would also feel responsible. I would never have dreamed of trying to parent children long-distance, but here I was with all the feelings of being a parent and there was nothing I could see to do to rectify this out-of-control situation.

As an interim solution I added extra trips to visit them to the POPlan. I reasoned that by increasing the frequency of seeing my parents in New York, I would provide them more direct attention and could also spend more of their "sunset" time with them. In one two-month interval I transported my body across our wide country eight times, and it was exhausting me. I wasn't that young myself, and I'd postponed some badly needed foot surgery. I couldn't imagine having my procedure and then walking around on crutches in the midst of my parents' "situation." Instead I hobbled up and down the corridors of hospitals and airport terminals that seemed to be growing increasingly long, ignoring my own medical needs.

Looking back to that time, I can see that once I'd taken on POP, I wasn't clear how to stay true to that commitment while also giving myself permission to take care of me. In my office I had seen too many POParents continue down this sacrificial path that I seemed to have found myself following. I even taught stress management seminars, so I knew for sure that if I didn't attend to myself, eventually I'd not be able to properly care for my folks. I would have to practice what I'd been preaching and walk the walk.

Then one day I got another phone call from Florence. When she'd taken my parents to their doctor visits, they'd instructed her to have me call as soon as possible. The bottom line was this: No help on nights and weekends was exhausting Jack and insufficient oversight for Lillian. Florence and the doctors were in agreement on this.

With that phone call, I saw that things were about to change again. In that moment, it was clear that they really might be leaving New York. My wish to end long-distance POParenting might now be granted. To realistically appraise the whole situation, I told myself: "Breathe! Breathe deeply enough to have sufficient oxygen go to your brain to think clearly." There was a lot to consider, and more things that I didn't know.

Dad and Mom were now eighty-seven years old and might easily live many more years; I certainly hoped so. Predictably, they would require increasing hours of help, not fewer. Our family

resources were hardly limitless, and reviewing them at this juncture was important since any decision would need to be grounded
in what was financially possible.

We had their LTC insurance benefits, which they were using at
the maximum number of hours already, their monthly Social Security checks, occasional music royalties, and the savings my parents had set aside for their later years. Plus, I had a small amount
of money saved, but I'd changed professions from attorney to
psychotherapist and I was just starting over in midlife to build my
new practice when POP had popped into my world. Although the
fear of running out of funds loomed and I wasn't certain how we'd
work it out, I knew I'd never give up on my commitment to do
POP.

Since everyone but Lillian and Jack agreed that my parents
needed more help, the simplest new POPlan would have to have
them accept additional hours of caregiving help on weekends and
nights. Such a plan afforded them continuity with their physicians,
Florence, their home, and beloved New York. But that plan also
had long-term downsides. I had to consider not only what my
parents would be willing to accept but also whether and how we
would afford their accelerating care needs.

Were my parents to "age in place"—that is, stay in their New
York home[2]—the number of hours of care required might soon
increase drastically, especially because of my mother's diagnosis of
Alzheimer's. Her illness would likely require full-time nursing
care eventually. Both of my parents might require live-in aides in
the future, and any hours of care, beyond what Florence already
provided, would all be our out-of-pocket expenses, uncovered by
LTC.

My other problem with this aging in place POPlan was that if
we continued living at this distance from each other, my capacity
to share my folks' sunset years would likely decrease. I might even
see them less often than I was now, with the added pressure on
me to bring in more income for their escalating care.

An alternative POPlan was that they move in with me. That
alternative had a lot of problems. I was gone all day at work and

my parents would need a caregiver to help them at least during those hours I was away, if not longer hours. That might have worked out, since they still had home health care benefits under their LTC policy, but several other factors made that option unworkable.

For one thing, a few months prior to Florence's call, when it seemed Jack and Lillian were forever settled in New York, I'd purchased a house that was not well suited for doing POP. You entered the house by either climbing forty-seven irregular steps in the back or thirty-eight even ones in the front. The first time Dad had gazed down at my amazing view after slowly huffing and puffing his way up those stairs, he'd said: "Terrific view! You should move!" There was nothing about the house's physical setting that would have worked well for my elderly parents. Likely they would have felt trapped because those daunting steps made going anywhere burdensome. The floor plan was compact and they would have had very limited privacy. There wasn't even a convenient place for a caregiver to sit down and rest.

Another reason moving in with me wasn't a good choice was because I didn't believe my parents and I would get along well living together while I was also parenting them. Many families find that when their roles become reversed doing POP, it's challenging to live together, especially when there have been decades of living far apart. I didn't think we'd operate as well under the same roof as separately after living a continent apart and observing my parents' generational "do it our own way" approach. Although we never had a formal discussion where any of us formally rejected this choice, Jack, Lillian, and I shared the understanding that the place I sought for them—even in a senior residence—would be their own home. They wouldn't be uncomfortably "borrowing" mine.

A third POPlan—and the most realistic—was that my parents would move into an attractive senior facility. In such an environment they could get sufficient "Florence-like" individual attention to be comfortable and protected while living more communally and maybe socially than in their New York apartment. They would get a chance to dine with others and could become involved in various social and recreational activities with their peers.

If they lived at a facility in New York City, I would again be relegated to long-distance POP. If they were going to leave their NYC apartment and have to face that loss, it would be just as easy to move them out to California as to some East Coast facility. Since most of their friends and living relatives had already moved to warmer climes or to be nearer to their kids, bringing my parents to my neighborhood wouldn't deprive them of their social support as it might have earlier on.

But the biggest advantage of their coming west to California was that we could become more involved in each others' everyday lives. Once I formulated this doable POPlan, I began to see them living in California. Lillian would be smiling and relaxed, a shawl lightly draped over her shoulders as she basked in our year-round warmth. Jack would be holding an iced tea in one hand, a music business weekly magazine in the other.

I imagined Dad and me at the end of my workday, talking like we'd done so long ago at the end of his. Then he'd recounted his exciting trips to the music business' Brill Building or news of another Frank Sinatra recording of one of his songs. I wondered what I'd recount to him about my day at work. In my mind's eye, more California sun and glasses of iced tea floated by. I could finally stop the bicoastal POParenting I'd never been comfortable with. This would be good, I found myself thinking.

I also was feeling proud of my ability to adapt to the needs of my parents' changing circumstances. I was congratulating myself on making good modifications to our initial POPlan and thoughtfully moving forward. I thought this new arrangement would give us everything we wanted. They could have their independence, a good climate, and a healthy life. We could be closer, making it easier to see each other and share our everyday lives again after so much time spent apart.

It wasn't long before the next phone call came in to burst my daydream. This time it was Dad who issued the bad news: "We're not coming. Your mother doesn't want to move to California." That was all he said.

THEIR STORY—MOM

I'd never thought much about death, and my religion of origin didn't provide a lot of guidance about an afterlife. And whenever I had considered the end of our lives, it was almost like Jack and I would age but stay pretty healthy, and eventually we'd sort of fade away in our apartment. One day we'd just be gone—off with our families in heaven. But like so many things these days, as I've gotten older, life has been turning out far differently than I ever imagined.

Since that first December when Jane started helping us out, she's been the one making more and more decisions for us. I didn't like that very much, but, since I couldn't focus very well and Jack clearly wasn't himself, it seemed that would have to do. I'd long been concerned that moving to California might mean my daughter would run my life, and I had always been apprehensive that my family would put me in a home for the aged someday. My siblings had done that to our mother when she had Parkinson's and Jane was just born.

When I came back home from the hospital after my horrible bout with pneumonia, I was surprised to see that the house had been cleaned from top to bottom. It was a very different place from how I'd left it. The fact that it was spotless again felt good. But by the same token, now there were also strangers who seemed to have taken over my home. In the beginning, these caregivers Jane had hired were there all the time, even when we slept. She'd insisted that I have a caregiver watch over me and that Jack have one too. I hated having so many people underfoot and watching me.

I also didn't like that these caregivers cost so much. They didn't have that much to do for Jack or me, so they sat around much of the day. Jane refused to let us be alone until I laid down the law and wouldn't let her get her way on that point. After a little while, Jack and I were able to work it out with Jane so we could have fewer people and more privacy in our home, which was a relief. We prevailed on her: no one there late nights or weekends.

That left one person helping us, Florence, whom I liked quite a bit. She had a good sense of people and wasn't too chatty, which I enjoyed. Florence just seemed to know when I'd be okay with her helping me and when I could do things on my own. She'd been there with Jack since the first day, and he was comfortable with her too. Florence had even worked for another family in our building, which I appreciated because she knew our maintenance staff as well.

Yet, despite our physical recoveries, our clean home, and attentive caregiver, and in spite of Jane's numerous visits, as time wore on, I watched my husband get more exhausted and agitated. He had never been this way. I was usually the more anxious one. It was disturbing to see him become so easily upset and so often. Psychiatry had been my refuge, while Jack had always been the consistent and calm one. When he needed to go see a psychiatrist for the first time in his life because he had ringing in his ears and, later on, obsessive and suicidal thoughts, I became panicked too. I feared that unless Jack straightened himself out, we might have to leave our home and move into some old-aged people's home or out to California. Jane had begun presenting these alternatives, but none of the options looked good to me.

Jane had been suggesting for a long time that Jack and I move out to California, her home state. It's very pretty out there and has been a lovely place for her to live and for us to come visit. But I don't picture myself as a "California gal." I've never surfed, and I'm not even sure I know what that involves. I've never been blond or even particularly suntanned. I am a New Yorker, and by choice. I moved here after Jack and I were married in 1941. We both harkened from Paterson, New Jersey, where we were born and raised, but we became dyed-in-the-wool New Yorkers. And we New Yorkers don't particularly crave the sun all day every day and don't necessarily want to know more about beaches and surfing.

I watched Jane very carefully in those early days of her caring for us. And it didn't seem that she wanted to put us anywhere we'd hate. In fact, as our daughter started visiting more often and doing more things for Jack and me, I saw a different sweetness come over her. Jane was sincere in wanting to listen to us. What we wanted or didn't want mattered to her, and I saw her struggling to find the best way to manage us and everything else she had on her plate. I eventually realized that she didn't have an agenda that involved controlling us and was trying to do the right thing. Much of her challenge was in figuring out how to protect Jack and me but still let us do things "our way," reprising Sinatra.

But I definitely didn't like what I was now being told. Our doctors had said it was "unmanageable" and "unacceptable" for Jack and me to stay in our home in New York without more caregiver help. Probably it would be best to move closer to Jane but I didn't like anything about what I was hearing. It was just too late in life to turn into a California girl. I wasn't going, so there.

YOUR STORY

The only predictable part about POP is continuous, unpredictable change. Make a plan and see. You'll need to get comfortable with change! If you want to thrive doing POP—or even survive it— you'll need at least two abilities: (a) discovering the changes in your parents' conditions or their environment and (b) responding quickly and wisely.

No one wants to learn that the existing POPlan—the one you worked so hard to make viable in all its details and that everyone likes—needs tweaking or, worse yet, total reconstruction. Your POP experience will benefit if and when you develop a more objective set of eyes and ears to detect changes in your parents' health and home, even if you're hesitant to see it. You *can* train yourself to become more scientific about the situation and to view more analytically any alterations in your parents' environment, physical body, and cognitive state.

If you're living at a distance, to some extent you'll need to rely on others to discover incremental changes, people who see your parents more regularly than you do. A professional caregiver, a doctor, a surrogate daughter, a GCM, and/or even a good neighbor will often be that person. You will want to keep those who are in your core POP group apprised of everyone's contact information and to schedule regular communications with them. Today's technology allows this to occur with ease, as you can copy family members on emails, reports, texts, or even Skype up the core POP group for a quick video conference call when needed.

Because of visits and/or your talking with those physically close to your parents, you will have updated, objective, and accurate information. Use it. You'll still need to regularly reexamine your current POPlan. Is it still viable today? Avoid the temptation to fix what's working well, but be willing to expand your ideas and fix what isn't working. Does your plan allow for your responding in a timely manner to observable shifts in your parents' circumstances? Are you "guilt-tripping" yourself into promising something more than you can give or are willing to follow through on?

To know the difference, look at your current plan from both sides of the POP equation. From your aging parents' perspective: Does the current POPlan provide me an optimal balance between self-sufficiency and safety? What, if anything, do I not like or find objectionable about the current arrangement? How might this situation be improved for my greater comfort or enjoyment? From you, the POParental perspective: Does the current POPlan take more out of you than you're comfortable giving—in terms of lost income, time with young grandchildren, or whatever else you value? What did you plan to spend your retirement resources on before POP happened? Does the arrangement give you the optimal balance between sufficiently protecting your parents from harm and your ability to "have a life"? What, if anything, do you not like about your current arrangement and how could it be improved for you?

If you want to do better than "survive" during your middle stages of POP—maybe even aspire to thrive—you will want to maximize some of your personal qualities that have shown themselves critical for your success in parenting and POParenting so far. At the least, you've needed your flexibility, your resiliency, and your ability to laugh at the small stuff in life. Now you can work to make these traits even more available to you as a POParent. You will find that focusing your intention and your attention on responding less automatically and allowing patience and outside-the-box thinking will add to your flexibility.

A powerful tool to do all of that and more is something I've referred to earlier and I call it "underreacting." By this I mean responding less automatically and less emotionally to setbacks, complications, and disappointments. It is a technique you can use over and over again during challenges in your POPcycle, when parenting your kids, and with your boss. By underreacting, you'll be able to lighten up and find humor in the midst of these challenges. When you and your parents can laugh more, everyone around you has more enjoyment.

You're right if you've decided that many things are out of your control during POP. You probably spent a lot of time and effort making a good POPlan. Perhaps it was a great plan. But if your mom or dad refuses to go along with it, what are your choices? If they refuse to see your point of view, it's simply not a great POPlan. Even if what you want to achieve is in your parents' best interest, how will you be able to impose it if they disagree or are at a distance?

Here, as in so many POPcycle challenges, the ideal POPlan for one family won't necessarily be the one for yours: one size does not fit all. You will need to listen to your parents' wishes as best you can and perhaps make some compromises. In some of your POP decisions, you may even need to do what POParents (and all parents) sometimes do—that is, take some protective action you believe is right even when it's contradictory to your parents' expressed desires. You've seen that I had to do that. Ultimately, you too may need to choose for them, especially if your parents are gravely incapacitated or otherwise not able to think clearly.

POParenting is not for the fainthearted or the easily discouraged. It's tricky because unlike when they parented you, you can't insist that your charges eat their vegetables or turn off the TV. But don't underestimate your powers of persuasion. Having chosen to be POP responsible, those powers to convince your parents may include the rightness of your position and the limitations of available finances—and, of course, your excellent reasoning. Or maybe it's really your love and concern that finally convinces your parents to follow your well-reasoned POPlan.

8

FINDING THE BEST FIT FOR OUR PARENTS' NEW HOME

MY STORY

In spite of the apparently unconditional nature of Dad's announcement, I knew that eventually I would bring my parents to California. It was the only responsible way for me to continue doing POP. I found I had an unusual sense of clarity, confidence, and determination in that moment.

My initial task was calming Mom down. I knew that when she was calmer, she would agree with what had become apparent to me, Florence, and their doctors—and, I presumed, to Dad as well. POParental rationality would need to take precedence over my parents' fears, concerns, or any other "good" excuses they might offer to avoid leaving home.

The near unanimity of opinion that moving to California was their wisest option fueled my feelings of competency and confidence. That was especially important because I would somehow have to override my parents' decision. By now, since the day I first confronted my father at his door and stepped up for POParenting, I also had plenty of practice utilizing those feelings. If this had been the first time, I might have been more reticent to challenge my parents or more concerned about their reactions. Perhaps I would have backed down.

I knew that I must not personalize any aggressive or hostile-sounding remarks I might receive when I was "forcing" people to do what they didn't want to do. Jack and Lillian didn't want to accept the truth that they needed more help than Florence could offer. But it was the truth nevertheless.

All things considered, that meant they would need to come live in California. The move wasn't only for Mom. I'd also seen Dad decline, getting weaker psychologically as well as physically because of the stress of caring for and gradually "losing" his fading beloved.

Lillian and I would talk many times before she was finally convinced. I knew I'd need to allow her to express herself as best she could for as long as she needed. My mother shared her fears about moving and how it evoked her long history of loss and abandonment. She told me of her concern that moving to California would alter her relationship with Dad and with me. I tried to reassure her that those changes could be wonderful, better than she could imagine, and I meant it. When she saw I was listening to her and, thankfully, she was cogent enough to get my message, she softened.

In spite of my own lingering hesitations, I reassured myself that their moving closer to me was the most intelligent, prudent, and loving POPlan for all concerned. All right! I'd just pack up their remaining stuff and we'd be on our way. Done with partial caregiver coverage and done with long-distance POParenting! At last!

As we all settled into the idea of the move becoming reality, I noticed an old twinkle return to Dad's eye. I hadn't seen it there for far too long. Jack was excited. He was relieved to be leaving the apartment and his heavy responsibilities in New York City. He looked forward to living closer to me after all these years and to my sharing his burden. In fact, Dad looked lighter and younger than I'd seen him in years. I thought I heard him whistling a tune that sounded like "California, Here I Come. . . ."[1]

If my parents had lived closer, I'd have first gone to scope out a bunch of places, narrowed my favorites to the top three or so and produced a short list for us to visit together. But since I wanted everything to be ready when they got off the long plane ride from New York, I had to make all the choices without any input from them. I had to figure out where they might like to live and that was not necessarily where I might have chosen were I choosing for me.

My goal was to find a facility where Lillian and Jack would do best—that is, feel at home, remain content, and maybe peaceably pass away some time in the very distant future. Their level of care already mandated some caregiving, so the purely Independent Living (IL) model for seniors was too unstructured for them. Nor did my folks yet require the more serious medical care available in a skilled nursing facility (SNF), where people need nurses.

Thus, my search became focused on finding them either an intimate, pretty homelike setting where they would get some personal attention—a six-bed board-and-care facility (B&C)—or an assisted-living facility (ALF), a larger structure where the senior residents live in their own apartments and share meals and activities.

Which type of setting would my parents fare better in—a small, six-bed B&C or a more populous and private ALF? In a B&C, residents live in a quaint converted home. Most of the time, each resident has a separate room, but all share meals, facilities such as a garden and a reading room, and much of their time together every day. Everything about a B&C, including the number of staff, residents, and size of the facility, is smaller.

An ALF sounded more like what my parents had known and loved in New York. I liked that. But I wondered if they might not prefer a more traditional California bungalow-type setting? Maybe they would enjoy living in a small B&C facility with just six bedrooms, where they could walk outside and read in the garden on a warm winter's day.

Either way, I had to imagine that I knew my parents' current tastes and preferences in location, type of residence, décor, and furnishings. Eventually I chose their residence and most of their furniture and furnishings as well. I bought many things to make it homey for them when they landed at their new place, since hauling a lot of their heavy items cross-country didn't prove to be a great idea. In a way, my "nesting process" before their arrival was another symbol of our role reversal—my doing for them the equivalent of what they'd done for me when they'd first brought me home, their newborn baby girl, all those years ago.

To narrow my search for the most suitable facility for my folks, I found help in the form of a geriatric placement agency. Happily, using their services didn't cost our family anything. Senior residences pay these firms, which function much like employment firms, offering interested families a menu of prospective residential choices. I chose this particular firm based upon recommendations I'd received and upon my intuitive sense of the woman who ran the company. I liked her questions, the way she posed them, and her professionalism. Like earlier on in the POPcycle when we'd needed a geriatric care manager (GCM), now it was the placement person who needed to understand a lot of background information concisely expressed to best counsel our family.

When the placement woman and I spoke, she reminded me of several significant criteria in settling aging parents into suitable facilities. Later, when I had to resettle each of my parents, I'd return to speak with her and I'd be reminded of the validity of her basic points. One key was to locate my parents near enough to my home and/or work so I would visit them frequently and oversee their care. Another key was the facility's having a good and caring staff—if possible, a stable staff of long-standing, so that Mom and Dad could avoid some of the separation feelings I anticipated they might have without faithful Florence.

Regarding proximity, I was well advised to be realistic. Longer distances do discourage even the most diligent and loving of POP-arents from visiting as often as they might like. When seeing my parents added a lot of drive time to my schedule at the end of a particularly challenging workday, I might end up not going. Moreover, if they lived close by me, visiting would be far more accessible. Not only could I be more casual and spontaneous but dropping in on my parents unexpectedly could prove useful. If some of my visits to my parents were "unplanned," I might obtain a more accurate view of how they really were or how the facility actually attended to them.

Many other factors came into the mix. I tried to put myself into the heads of my parents. What did Mom and Dad like to do? Who did they wish to get to know? How did they spend their time? What would Jack most enjoy in a new home? He had become far more introverted than my memory of him when we were both so much younger. What did he like? Unless I turned the radio or stereo on, he rarely listened to music in New York. Maybe he just enjoyed the quiet? Dad read a lot and watched his TV shows. *Jeopardy* and *The Tonight Show* were his favorites. He ate, did some stretching at home, meditated, and talked to Mom and to me. That's basically what I'd seen when I'd visited in New York, and I expected he'd be similarly quiet once he'd settled into the West Coast lifestyle.

Lillian was far more outgoing. She had previously enjoyed crossword puzzles, listening to music, taking drives through Central Park and watching plays. Still beautiful at age eighty-seven, she could be gracious and friendly with others. Much of the time she still appeared engaged and very affable. But she could become hostile, haughty, demanding, aggressive, and unreasonable— sometimes without any apparent triggering events. I suspected Mom's discovering that her mind was increasingly beyond her control resulted in much of her frustration and bad behavior. Although I sympathized with her pain, her condition made it challenging to predict which type of senior facility might be best.

During our New York POP years, I came to witness Lillian's dementia manifest in volatile temper tantrums manifested in pinching, punching, bullying, demeaning, and scratching Dad. She repeatedly threatened him that she'd jump from her fourteenth-story bedroom window. It was painful to watch. Dad had become frailer and never acted aggressively with her. On a few occasions when Mom's disorders would overcome her, I had to intervene between my parents. As the emerging disciplinarian, it

was now becoming my job to set the limits of my parents' acceptable conduct. That definitely felt like role reversal gone wild.

So far, most of Mom's aggressiveness had been directed at
Dad, but I wondered if she might act out with others in her new
place, particularly when the dementia would further take her over.
Telling the placement professional this history was important so
we could find a facility that would most suit all my parents' needs,
emotional, physical, and mental.

I had concerns about placing them in a smaller B&C facility
with my mother's history of being a difficult patient. I'd seen her
blow through a series of hard-core veteran caregivers in those
early 24/7 care days in New York. I questioned how soon her
fellow residents and the small number of caregivers in any B&C
might become a problem for Lillian. I kept returning to the notion
that such an intimate setting as six beds could provide too many
opportunities for Mom to become upset and/or to upset others.

With this in mind, I turned my sights to locating a serene, nice-
looking larger ALF. With the list of ten in hand that my placement
professional had given me, I drove from one to the next, checking
out all of them. None proved quite right for Lillian and Jack.
Nonetheless, while visiting one on my list, someone there recommended an eleventh place that I liked immediately.

This ALF seemed to offer the right blend of serenity and activity and was geographically pretty attractive in its proximity to my
home and work. And, as I would soon discover, it had the additional element I sought: a caring and longtime staff. I respected
the people I talked with who worked there and liked their attitude
toward "their" people. The staff I met seemed genuinely interested in expanding the quality of life, not just babysitting the residents.

The more I heard about this independently owned and operated ALF, the better it sounded. Mom and Dad would be provided
much on-site in terms of exercise, recreation, holiday celebrations,
and even health monitoring. A van took interested residents daily
to the local mall for shopping, banking, and sundry errands. I even

saw other transplanted New Yorkers, whom I imagined might become friends with my parents.

To do my due diligence, I visited the facility a number of times. I went at different times of day. I tasted the food, smelled around a lot, and asked a lot of questions. I wandered about, talked to the residents, their families, and to more of the staff. I questioned people I knew in the community about the facility. It all sounded quite fine.

Although I went about the tasks methodically and as unemotionally as I could, I mistakenly thought I'd become inured to the sadness and other emotions that got stirred up while I looked for a place for my own parents. This was how they would end up living their final days. I guess I'd convinced myself that my clarity about the decision to move them to California and my extensive professional background would "simplify" my feelings.

I soon found that choosing a residence for my own parents was very different from visiting similar facilities for my patients. Even walking into the first senior residence felt emotionally wrenching for me as I contemplated what it meant to be "institutionalizing" my own Mom and Dad. I plagued myself with unanswerable questions about where I would end up. What would it be like when my turn to move out of my home came?

POP provided me the chance to ask myself questions about how I wanted to age. There was longevity in my family on both sides. I began to recount the list of my aunts and uncles who lived into their nineties. Even my maternal grandmother with Parkinson's had lived until seventy-eight, and that was over fifty years ago! My relatives had been healthy people with little obvious dementia and few physical disturbances. I could see that being ill while old could deplete much of the joy of being alive. Looking down the road ahead, I recommitted to my own healthy living.

It would be a good life for them, I assured myself. I made the decision and filled out the application on their behalf. Before I could seal the deal, I needed my parents to be accepted by the AL. I understood that different facilities have varying requirements, and I was relieved and thankful when they told me my parents met theirs.

The apartment I chose for them had a small balcony where Mom and Dad could sit on comfortable patio chairs with blankets and gaze over magnificent oak trees. Or so I envisioned. Next, I went around town furnishing their new home, right down to purchasing their favorite toothpaste and bedside books. I so wanted it to feel like home when they got there after their long plane ride and, more importantly, leaving their home in New York.

I was elated that I had found a suitable and attractive place for Jack and Lillian. It was the answer to my POP prayers that we could finally end our long-distance POParenting. However, as their move became a reality and was actually upon us, I was surprised to discover that I had some mixed feelings that weren't all positive. On the one hand, I was reassured that I could better monitor my parents' well-being from up close. But on the other, I felt clueless about how it would be to have them living so close and, as a result, I became anxious.

When I get anxious, my mind starts feeding me questions. How would we all do living in such close proximity at this time in our POPcycle? How often would I see them: once a week or every day? Would they or I want visits to be more frequent? How would I find them decent physicians? Would I take them to their every dentist and doctor appointment? And if so, how would I afford the time? Would they even want that? How would they get to the drug store to buy toothpaste? Or would that task and so many more now become mine?

I was full of unknown speculation and unanswerable questions. I even had some fears that, doing POP up close and personal, I might "fail." Although I intellectually knew that time would answer all these questions, sometimes it was particularly difficult to replace my anxiety with the faith in myself and the universe's goodness I usually experience.

Most of the time I was able to use my thoughts constructively—to support me in dealing with knotty POP challenges such as unnerving instances of role reversal. I defined those as when I was "being the grown-up" instead of the child in my relationship with my parents. At this stage of our POPcycle, being the parent meant taking care of all the physical details of finding their new place and helping them settle in, much like when they'd taken me to settle into summer camp or college.

Being the POParent also involved securing a solid emotional base for my aging folks to lean on. One way I was seeing I could use this role reversal to all of our benefits was to remember what I had craved from parents when I'd been the child—and then shower it on them. I'd wanted my parents' unconditional love, acceptance, permission to lean on them without shame, and a spiritual rootedness. And whether or not they'd been able to give me all of that back when I was young, I saw this as my chance to offer those very qualities to them, now that I was being the grown-up.

There were other times when I was less the consummate adult, times my mind created unnecessary problems for me. For example, when I attributed a fearful meaning to this stage of the POPcycle, I found myself succumbing to a deep sense of loss. Similarly, I'd make myself upset when I obsessed over thoughts of my onetime protectors needing a protected environment or my beloved parents descending a winding road toward increasing attendants and then death.

Lawyer Jane would even try to argue me out of my sinking sadness. I tried to convince myself it wasn't logical to be upset now, since I'd long accepted that my folks needed a fair amount of help from Florence, and now they just needed more. Psychotherapist Jane jumped in and encouraged me to observe my fearful and sad thoughts, rather than allow myself to get drawn into or paralyzed by them. Sometimes that was hard to do, since my feelings seemed to want to "run me."

POParenting required me to pull myself back into the present as quickly as I could because it was in that authentic present—and without drama—that I made my most sensible and wise decisions. And right now, my parents were not leaving the planet or me but just New York, and they needed to live in a place precisely like the one I'd worked so hard to find.

Doing POP is, by definition, bittersweet. My folks seemed so vulnerable now, not the invincible figures they'd been years before, when they'd been "the parents." I was POParenting older parents whose aging genetically programmed them to become less capable of independence and ultimately more childlike. This is strikingly opposite to the experience of parenting children, who are genetically programmed to do the opposite—they become more .independent and less infantile. When we launch the children we've raised and fallen in love with, we're shipping them off to (presumably) bright, shiny careers, schools, and marriages to fulfill what they learned originally when they were with us. But when we launch our beloved parents, we're sending them off to apparent emptiness and the big unknown.

Anticipating their moving closer, I recognized that proximity would also allow me to observe my parents' day-to-day declines. It seemed to make the time we had left together especially poignant. None of these times could ever be recaptured, but I most often noticed the bittersweet taste when my parents seemed most like their old selves again. It was as if I could see through the old people they'd become to the individuals I used to know. Those remembered parents sometimes seemed more real than the aged couple in front of me.

In the early 2000s I trained under the direction of Dr. Martin Seligman and his expert network of researchers and clinicians I named the "Happiness Scientists."[2] Their rigorous studies validated some conclusions I'd also reached while working with patients in my office. Doing certain practices regularly and repetitively can and will retrain a brain's connections. I learned that we can expand our capacity for real joy in life by consistently engaging in three activities—being grateful, granting forgiveness, and savoring the good in our lives. As a result of doing so, we can reset the level of our "happiness thermostat," that internal mechanism that operates to regulate our emotions much like a thermostat regulates the temperature in our homes. One thermostat raises our environmental temperature and the other our internal happiness level. It was apparently up to me to move that dial, and I could indeed raise it!

Once Mom and Dad moved into my world in California, I reminded myself that I could—and probably should—practice this happiness formula for myself specifically in relation to doing POP. On a daily basis, I made the determined practice to invoke all three: gratitude for having them as my parents and being able to share that appreciation by joyously POParenting; forgiving my parents, and myself, mainly for being human; and delighting in the gift of this moment. I promised myself to focus on the sweet side of the bittersweet, savor the present and its many good times while doing POP.

While not denying my real sadness, especially when I anticipated the future of our POPcycle, I didn't see much utility in bathing in that grief either. I would remind myself: Live in the present, Jane! Your parents are very much alive! After thirty-five years of living apart, I now had the chance to become closer and more loving with my family and to accentuate the positive in all of that would add to its sweetness.

The three of us needed me to be enthusiastic and to share with Jack and Lillian how attractive the move and their new place would be for them. I'd be no good for any of us if I continued to concentrate my thoughts on their "inevitable descent" or talk about this upcoming phase as "institutionalizing" my folks. Those words sounded very dramatic but didn't really represent my truth.

Instead, I could more accurately and helpfully coach myself by applying a tool from cognitive research called "reframing" my thinking. Reframing involves examining our thoughts and noticing how else we might think about the same topic, perhaps more neutrally and less emotionally. What I'd been telling myself was that moving them to the ALF was "putting them in an institution." When I applied the tool of reframing, I could envision that same activity as "picking out my parents' next home." How much more positively I could—and did—feel, and how much more energized I was to complete the task, with that new point of view!

Simply shifting my way of thinking about their move helped quite a bit. Afterward, I was far more comfortable settling my parents in, even making decorating choices for them with more ease and confidence. Reframing became a reliable technique and POP coaching tool that I was happy to teach so many of my clients. And, it was a tool I would return to myself often during my time of POParenting, especially when I found myself feeling stuck in repetitive unwanted feelings.

The ALF I chose for Mom and Dad was only a few short miles from my home. The eucalyptus trees just outside their patio provided beauty, shade, and a distinctive aroma I've come to associate with Southern California. Downstairs, the food smelled great and tasted even better. Mom would soon be looking forward to a sitting yoga class while Dad would enjoy reading undisturbed in the quiet library.

I wondered: "Is there a minimum age to move in?"

YOUR STORY

Most families will have many options for elderly parents to safely live out their final days. If your parents need to move from their current location, hopefully you can choose a place that will remain a viable residence through the course of their illnesses and declines so you can avoid moving them multiple times. Multiple moves add to everyone's turmoil and they present particular challenges for those with cognitive limitations. Moving away from familiar settings is disorienting and sometimes appear to trigger the final decline and death of seniors. Moving from home to an ALF to one SNF after another, as my mom's conditions eventually required were traumatic each time. It's stressful for any of us to have to move our stuff and ourselves from our home, and then to readjust and have to learn many new things. But for seniors with dementia, it is best if we can POPlan in advance for as few moves as possible.

It should come as no surprise that most Americans over fifty would prefer to remain living in their own home than have to move. My parents did, and yours may too. Certainly, one reason people don't want to move involves the series of upsets associated with it: the loss of familiar people, places, and activities and the anxiety of the unknown ahead. Experts claim that moving is one of the highest stressors in life. It's also hard physical work to prepare, sort, pack up, cart, haul, unpack, and replace things in new places. If moving is hard on a healthy adult, you can only imagine how much more traumatic it might be to your parents. They rarely have the mental or physical energy, stamina, and level of recall that younger people do.

Essentially, your POP choice comes down to three approaches: aging in place; moving to a relative's home, or choosing a senior "institutional living" facility. None of these is inherently superior to any other. Each type of living experience is very different, and each has its advantages and disadvantages. In deciding, you face the uncertainty of not knowing the number of years your parents have left. If you have limited resources—and who doesn't—you'll need to consider price as you look over these alternatives. Other costs, such as your own emotional, physical, or cultural demands, may be even harder to calculate.

If your parents want to "age in place" (stay in their home with extra measures taken to protect them) and your TEAM POP agrees they can do so without much apparent risk, that may be your best option. There are some great advantages for your parents if they can stay living where they've resided for a long time. By staying where they have long actively engaged in life and everything is familiar, your parents may enjoy stability and community that are irreplaceable. Having to adjust to a new home, to new neighbors, new routines, and to so much else that is unknown can be taxing at any age. During their senior years, such a move can be overwhelming.

But neither should you underestimate how upsetting, sad, or depleting moving your parents may be for you. Some of you, like me, will be packing up homes where you grew up. During this process you may find yourself caught up in nostalgia and other emotional memory jogging. It may bring tears to your eyes to watch your sweet, maybe shorter, loved ones go to their favorite haunt together one last time. I choked up watching Jack and Lillian at their local deli savoring their last New York corned beef sandwiches on corn rye with sour pickles. Seeing your parents leave behind friends or siblings with whom they shared both happy and tougher times, knowing they'll never see each other again, can wrench you apart. Many of these moments can be avoided if your parents stay in their home.

Should your parents be able to age in place, you will find a growing industry to help you create in-home environments that support staying at home as a decent and safe alternative to institutional life. Unlike the POParents who will need to find a new setting, your challenges will be to help make your parents' current housing become even better. If you can avoid having your parents move late in life, their successfully aging in place will also necessitate more work for you. You may need to make modifications to their environment so they can access sufficient safety and hygiene methods as well as obtain good nutrition, stimulation, and social interaction. Then you will also need to see that those things actually are happening and, later, also check that they are working well.

Those who advocate aging in place remind us that many senior parents can stay happily and safely living in their homes, even living alone, *provided* certain modifications are made and/or certain technology is available. Others point out that aging in place may also require assistance from occasional or full-time help. If one or both of your parents served in the US military, they may qualify for a program called Aid and Attendance (A&A) Pension. It provides benefits for veterans and their surviving spouses who need another person to regularly attend and assist the person in eating, bathing, dressing, and undressing, or taking care of the needs of nature.[3]

Another group of modern geriatric professionals, certified aging-in-place specialists (CAPS), is available to help your parents remain at home. Their offerings can be particularly useful if your parents' need for modifications is a result of a traumatic event (usually a fall) or a more progressive decline in their function or mobility.

Falling is the leading cause of injurious events to older people. The two major goals of suggested home modifications are to prevent falls and to allow seniors better access to their possessions and daily activities. Some repairs involve taking steps that are as simple and inexpensive as removing clutter and dangerous throw rugs. Other modifications may include installing handheld flexible shower heads, grab bars, and nonskid flooring in appropriate locations. Increasing lighting, railings, and accessible light switches near stairs are also often recommended measures. In general, adding more light to the environment of our seniors is very helpful—whether by replacing bulbs with stronger ones or adding additional lighting and lamps.

Other modifications may be costlier and require hiring a skilled person, perhaps a contractor, electrician, plumber, or a handyman. You may need help if you wish to create sliding shelves and drawers, build walk-in closets and showers, or widen entryways or build ramps for wheelchair access. Your out-of-pocket cost for these installations is likely to be well worth the long-term savings to life, limb, and everyone's stress levels. Perhaps there is also a program where you live that will help pay for such fixes.

Technology's contributions to your parents' ability to age in place grow with every moment. Smart houses are being developed to address the variety of hazards associated with the cognitive and physical declines of older adults. "Elder cams" run on the same surveillance premise that "nanny cams" offer concerned parents watching their children. Even now, apps on your smartphone can allow you or your parents' keyless entry and cashless payments for needed POP items. In all likelihood, all sorts of new tech tools will come along to help your parents remain as independent as possible in their own dwelling.

If your parents are fifty-five or older and meet certain conditions, they may be eligible to stay living in their community and receive comprehensive care at home rather than in a skilled nursing home under a federal program entitled Program of All-Inclusive Care for the Elderly (PACE).[4] This began as a pilot project and because it was so well received, it has been expanded to many American communities. Over time, we may see other programs that support aging in place becoming even more accessible.

But like the other options, aging in place has its disadvantages too. There is a toll that having your parents' stay in their home may take on you. As I have said, when my parents were aging in place, I had numerous long-distance POParenting concerns and distressing weekends until their conditions left our family without that option. Aging in place is complicated when all the adult children (or the only child) live at a distance or when those who live close by are already occupied caring for their children, homes, jobs, and lives.

Another problem with your parents remaining at home is the danger of their becoming socially isolated there. As your parents age, several factors coalesce to make this period a potentially lonely one. If your parents no longer go out to a job or senior day care, they may spend many days or much of every day sitting alone in their homes, having no contact with other people. Your parents' closest friends and relatives may have died, moved, or divorced. Now there may be few if any of them left in the neighborhood. As caring POParents, we cannot overlook the growing data of the great toll loneliness has on our isolated seniors and the real advantages of some well-cooked meals spent in the company of peers.

Your parents' diminished senses of sight, smell, hearing, and/or taste may affect their interest in and enjoyment of other people's company. Being in pain or having little energy similarly makes socializing a strain. Some of your parents will even experience shame or embarrassment if they have become forgetful or can't easily learn new things. All of this has the potential to have your parents further insulate themselves and remain within the so-called safety inside their homes.

At this point in their development your parents may have little inclination to leave home to meet new people or make new friends. If they remain living in their own home, your parents are likely to relate to fewer and fewer people and live in a smaller and smaller world over time. Exceptions exist and perhaps your mother attending her years-long Tuesday-night canasta game with "the girls" might be one. Or something unexpected and wonderful may happen in their lives, like your parents becoming best friends with a couple who happened to be seated near them in a restaurant. However, your parents will likely have diminishing social support and engagement if they age in place.

A part of your POParenting responsibilities will be to discover how to encourage your parents to get out of their homes, hang out with their friends, and attend activities they enjoy. It is part of your job to be keen to symptoms that may look like depression. Loneliness and isolation can lead to clinical depression and even suicide. If they will allow you to, your finding interesting local activities or arranging the equivalent of senior "playdates" might just lift your parents' spirits.

If your parents can stay in their home, you may be able to undermine some of this loneliness by staying in better communication with your parents, maybe better than I was. Skype, the internet, FaceTime, and the many other communication developments since my parents were long distance can help you mitigate the potential danger of your parents becoming too cut off. Sharing family events they cannot attend and keeping up with their grandchildren on the computer can bring your parents immediate pleasure and keep them involved in your life and vice versa.

The second major approach for where your parents can age comfortably is for you or your siblings to offer them a place to live in one of your homes. If you're thinking you might be willing to step up for that, stop and ask yourself: is it optimal to bring my parents to live in my home? And if your answer is a clear "no," whether immediately or after much soul-searching, consider whether your sister or brother's home would be any better. If you or your siblings answer "yes," you will need to assess whose home would be best for your parents and why. If you and your siblings have responded affirmatively, all of you should read these next paragraphs carefully. If your answer is "no," for all your homes, you will need another alternative altogether and can read below about institutional options.

But just because you and your parents *can* make it work, to bring an aging and/or ill, disabled, and demented parent into your home doesn't mean it's really the best choice for any of you. You need to discover if POParenting in your home is viable for you and whether it is the optimal place for your parents over the long haul. Realistically evaluate your parents' current and imminent needs. You may think you can watch your parents more carefully if they live in your home than in theirs or in a residence but maybe not. I believe it is crucial to search your heart and mind before you answer, perhaps in the way you did before deciding to bring a child into your home.

Analyze all the elements involved before committing to a potentially life-altering transition for everyone living in your home. Look at the many different aspects of your current life, including your employment, relationship with your spouse, your health, and your home's configuration. Recall your long-standing history with your parents and how you've all fared more recently together.

If you work full-time or part-time, would you have to sacrifice your job or its benefits to care for the parents in your home? What if your parents' disabilities eventually require two to three aides to transfer them from their beds to the bathroom commode, as my Mom did, toward her end? If your parents' cognitive declines require increasing hours of professional care or even more care-givers, would your home still be optimal or even an acceptable location? Would that be affordable in your home or would you need to move your parents again?

Consult a variety of family caregiver support programs, such as AARP and other organizations focused on family caregivers and their special needs. Find out the costs, financial and emotional, and learn about the benefits. Talk with others who brought their parents into their homes and listen carefully to what they have to share. Go online to the POP website and communicate with other POParents who are doing that in real time at the POP website, www.ParentingOurParents.org. You may be exposing yourself and your family to the rigors of living with chronic disease and/or dementia. Hearing details of how doing that affected other families may provide you with very useful insights. Even if your spouse, your children, and your siblings all believe that "everything will be just fine and we'll help too," listen carefully to your own wisdom!

As you assess your own limitations and those of your parents, you want to think in detail and be alert to the most likely possibilities. For example, is there enough security in your home for your dad with Alzheimer's? Such patients often wander off without securely locked exits. How will your parents negotiate the steps in your home if they need a walker and have to go to the bathroom in the middle of the night? Will they be waking you?

Can your marriage survive if it's already in a stressed state and your parents move in along with your "boomerang" adult children? If everyone ordinarily is away from 8 a.m. until after dark, can your parents prepare their own lunches, go to their doctors unaided, and be alone all day? Will they need a caregiver for some hours in your house? Will you be able to "hold your head up" in your family if you refuse the traditional dictates of your culture that "require" you to bring your parents into your home?

If no relative's home is right for your aging parents, where will you and your family look next? Your third approach for today's senior residences is the wide range of attractive institutional options. Although the term "institutional life" may sound off-putting, like you'd be shipping your parents to the back ward of some old, dank hospital in the 1950s, quite the opposite is true today. At one end of the spectrum, some institutions are simply private apartments in buildings or communities with other seniors. At the other end are locked settings where the residents' mobility and care are provided by staff.

What type of out-of-home experience is most suitable for your parents? The first step, which you've already begun, is to become clear about what level of care your parents require for their safety. Since you hardly want to see them as weak or needy, beware not to underestimate the extent of your parents' disabilities or their need for assistance.

The institutional setting for seniors with the fewest needs is termed IL.[5] These facilities permit "as needed" caregiving services to be added to your parents' bill or allow POParents to hire outside assistance. If your parents were able to care for themselves fairly well in their own home, this might be a good choice. However, if they need more care or you envision that happening in their near future, your parents may be better off living at the next level of caregiving, an ALF and avoiding the necessity for multiple moves.

Some ALFs and IL facilities have very specific restrictions. Most won't admit a resident who has a gastric feeding tube and require a resident to be able to evacuate the building without assistance in case of an emergency. Some offer flexibility by having different levels of care provided residents on different floors in a single building. If your parents become more needy, one or both of them can stay in the same facility but move to a different floor. This allows for continuity in location and staffing as well as permitting couples to have much contact in spite of being at different levels of aging. A Continuing Care Retirement Community (CCRC) is an option that offers families a contract that allows for continuity of residents at a single location during the entire POP-cycle, with fluidity in the resident's housing and needed nursing care.

Your TEAM POP can meet to clarify and prioritize the desired characteristics of the new residence that meet your parents' specific needs and desires. You can use a POP Family Coach to help you and your parents sort out the various choices and parameters of this critical decision and help you be better equipped to find precisely what you're looking for and know when you've found it. You'll also need to check out which facilities have space available and what is affordable for your family. Cleanliness, the number of residents, proximity to family, privacy, and accessibility to your parents' doctors, churches, transportation, and stores are certainly likely to be relevant features in your evaluation. It will be helpful for you to consider the attractiveness of the setting; size of the rooms, closets, and bathrooms; the extent of the recreational activities; the attention you observe that is given the residents by staff; and, of course, the quality of the food.

You will want to inquire about their professional people. I liked to hear that the staff remained working at a facility for a long time, since that longevity probably represented satisfied employees and my parents could feel assured that the staff would be there with them over time. In some states, such as California, senior facilities are required to maintain and make available to consumers a book in which all problem situations and their fixes are noted. If you have that advantage, you can look at any remarks or history and are likely to find it highly instructive. You can see if governmental authorities issued any orders or negative reports and ask lots of relevant questions. Consider moving on if you're not okay with their answers.

Your POP role will be evaluating the alternatives and making your parents' transition as seamless as possible. It will begin with your helping them accept that their leaving home is necessary and end after you've settled them into their new home. As you begin to look at these residences, you will develop a nose—often literally—for one that is likely to work best for your parents. And where else can you go to find your parents' new home? Fortunately, there are lots of methods to locate senior living facilities. Word-of-mouth, online searches, governmental reports, and professional referrals can each prove helpful to you. Increasingly, online entities provide their take on what will be good for your family, but beware that many websites are commercially sponsored or supported.

Your parents may protest and not like your choice. They may believe and wish you to believe they need less attention than is really warranted. Many will be concerned about the cost of all of this. Maybe your parents are embarrassed at the loss of some of their faculties or mistakenly see that as a weakness to be hidden. I always recommend that you treat your parents' aging limitations with respect and kindness and that you honor your parents' intelligence even in their last days. However, if your dad repeatedly can't remember to turn off the water when he runs his bathtub, you will need a facility that makes sure that happens, either by requiring you to hire additional help or providing it.

Professional placement agencies, such as the one I used, are another link in the geriatric service industry. They will need to interview you or your family's representative and maybe your parents as well. They will be discovering your requirements and hearing your preferences. After that, they will generate a list of maybe ten facilities for you to visit. Similar to how employment agencies work, their services are generally paid for by the residential facilities and are therefore complementary to the families. They can help you see where on the POPcycle your aging loved ones really are; clarify your priorities; and provide up-to-date information on charges, availability, and facility requirements.

As with other "real estate" decisions, the three watchwords for your POP housing choice may be location, location, location. When you start visiting your parents often, it will be clear why it's easiest to do POP locally when they live close by. It also might be advantageous to find a facility near to a freeway or on your route to work. Proximity to public transportation for your parents who may not drive can also be wise.

Our government regulates today's senior facilities. Most you will find are respectable and some are so elegant, you'd bet you were in a boutique hotel. Nonetheless, there are still some institutions that have significant problems that can pose a concern for POP families. How will you be able to know which is which?

In addition to the ways already suggested to check out facilities, you now have two specific websites to help you learn about their defects and governmental inspections. The Centers for Medicare and Medicaid Services surveys and certifies the nation's roughly fifteen thousand nursing homes. It has made available online the full text of reports that nursing home inspectors have filed for each of these facilities, a step many have urged for years. By going to https://www.medicare.gov and navigating your way to Nursing Home Compare, you can access this useful data. You can also do POP research at http://projects.propublica.org/nursing-homes, a website set up by a nonprofit organization of journalists. This site allows you to specifically discover nursing home defects in a simple, state-by-state manner.

There are always scary stories when people with some vulnerability, like our elderly loved ones, are living in institutional settings. And you must always stay vigilant when your parents are living in such places, but few are anything like what my mother had dreaded from the 1940s and 1950s. These days, most senior residential facilities pose few hazards and the majority of people who live there are grateful for the companionship, care, and activities afforded them in these residences.

9

DEALING WITH ALL
OUR PARENTS' STUFF

MY STORY

Laughter has always served me well. When I was confronting my toughest POP challenges, I needed to rely on humor the most. Sometimes when I was doing some aspect of POParenting with Lillian and Jack, comedy routines I remembered from my childhood would come back to me, seemingly unbidden. At precisely the moment I needed to begin examining all my parents' worldly possessions and decide what to do with them, a classic George Carlin monologue appeared. In it, he had warned us of people becoming dominated by their "stuff."

Carlin claimed that, without being aware of it, we could end up making all our life decisions based upon our stuff. We could use our stuff as the basis to choose our homes ("looks like a good place to put our stuff"), know when it's moving time ("we have too much stuff; we'd better move on") and even pick our line of work ("that's the way we get to buy more stuff"). I particularly loved the part where he pointed out the vast divide between other people's so-called garbage—although he used a different word for it—and our own valuable things.

Carlin's routine not only made me laugh (one of my "life tools" and favorite POP coaching tools) but also made me think about how best to manage my parents' lifelong collection of possessions. Transporting them and their things to California was an enormous undertaking. For a fully functioning forty-year-old who's lived in a small apartment for only a few years, relocating across town can be taxing. Moving and/or disposing of everything two eighty-seven-year-olds had ever acquired and schlepping them and their remaining things across the country was, to put it mildly, huge. When I reminded myself that my parents would never return here, that awesome thought added even more weight to the impending drama I was primed to experience.

As was my way, I made a list. That helped me keep myself organized and on target. I loved making lists because I loved checking things off. Completing this list was particularly satisfying, since, as I crossed off items, it meant we were that much closer to getting them settled in their new home.

The first thing on my list was to prepare Mom and Dad physically and emotionally for what was ahead. My goal was a bit delicate. I wished to enroll them in the excitement and momentum of their move without getting them fatigued or overwhelmed. I explained to my folks the general scenario.

1. Jane looks over all of Mom and Dad's things to get a good picture of the overall situation.
2. Jane sorts their possessions into categories—things they'd need on the plane or immediately when they arrived in California; things I'd ship to their new home; items to be given away; larger or more expensive pieces of furniture, antiques, or nonmemorabilia I would sell.
3. Jane consults as appropriate with Mom and Dad on these categories so they don't feel they're losing control over their stuff.
4. Jane packs the items to be shipped (with some "manpower" help), organizes the giveaways and arranges to sell the valuables.

5. Jane ships, gives away, and sells those things.
6. We three fly to Los Angeles together.

I explained my list, that we could bring much of their everyday clothing by air and that they'd be able to take their treasured and familiar things to their new place. Then I asked if they had any questions, but they didn't. I sensed their appreciation that this was a big job and they had confidence I would do it well. That felt good.

Later, when the apartment was emptied of all my parents' possessions, I would write another list. That second list was for me to begin hiring people to clean, paint, and refresh an apartment that hadn't been well maintained for many years. It had been a decade, maybe two, since Mom had been willing to allow anyone in from the building to fix the plaster and paint. As a result of these years of neglect, the metal screening behind the plaster, ordinarily several layers below the paint, had become bare and exposed to view. It was a bizarre contrast to look up from the elegant antiques in my parents' beautifully decorated home to the ceiling and see Sheetrock.

Eventually, I hired a real estate agent to rent or sell "their" apartment. Years before POP began, my folks had transferred their interest in the apartment to me as part of their estate planning. Technically it had become my apartment back then, but no matter what the ownership papers said, it always felt like my parents' place to me. Like so many of their generation, my parents' apartment had been their major life investment. By age forty-seven, Jack had worked hard to achieve some commercial success in the music business and was finally in a position to purchase (along with a little financial backing from his relatives) a home for "his girls," as he called Mom and me in those pre–women's liberation days.

My folks had been very proud to be able to buy their home and fulfill the American Dream.[1] And what an American Dream they'd found! Our Manhattan high-rise was beautiful! It was erected on the site of a lavish mansion and rose twenty-two stories high, above lush Central Park. The architect had won awards for his vision of our lobby, which retained the antique marble columns and fountain from the former building and integrated them with the ultramodern glass doors and windows of the new one.

I'd been in seventh grade when the building was in construction. The three of us eagerly visited each Saturday, excited to discover what the workers had accomplished during the previous week. Had they put up the new walls yet or installed the air conditioners? Was the carpeting laid, and how did it look? Later on, after we'd moved in, my friends and I watched a major motion picture, *Butterfield 8*, being filmed in our lobby. We were preteen girls and tried to imitate Elizabeth Taylor's sultry walk in her Oscar-winning performance, probably providing much humor for the building staff looking on.

Decades later, when Mom had become old and was bored being in the apartment, she would ask Florence or me to take her down to sit in that lobby, where she enjoyed chatting with her neighbors and our building's workers. Now I wondered if they'd found her amusing too. So many memories!

As I started taking the paintings off their walls, sorting and packing up my parents' possessions, I felt an odd sense of comfort. For forty-two years that apartment had been my parents' home. Originally, it had been my home base too. I'd only lived there for five years, back in the late 1950s and early 1960s, but a piece of me always considered it my home. Since my parents had stayed on there after I'd gone on to college, law school, and other pursuits, even after I'd developed my life in California, their apartment had remained my historic domicile.

We had been the only family to have lived in and loved inside those apartment walls. If there were secrets pressed into the recesses of those peeling plaster walls, they were our family's secrets. I wondered what those walls would have revealed, had they been able to speak. The familiarity of working among their things seemed to ground me at the time when what lay ahead seemed so unknown and shifting. I knew my focus should remain on completing these tasks, but my emotions sometimes proved demanding and distracted me. My lists were organized, but my feelings were dizzying and all over the map.

Some days I'd arrive ready to work on my self-assigned tasks only to discover that Mom and Dad had more pressing things for me to do from their perspective. Most of the time, I'd stop and divert from my lists because I felt I should attend to something they felt was more immediate. Other times I could only work for a limited amount of time because my emotions did take hold of me, almost weighing me down. As I sorted through their boxes of life treasures, I felt like I was watching a soap opera. But the characters weren't strangers; they were the nearest and dearest members of my family. I would unearth photos of my family or myself when we were all younger, and reminiscences would suddenly be triggered and carry me off into the past.

Now that I was seeing and handling all their stuff, I was surprised at how much I'd never been aware of. Could it be that I really knew very little about these two people? I remember having a momentary epiphany, childlike in its simplistic nature: my parents were people with lives before I knew them, before they even knew each other. They'd had lives before—and aside—from being *my parents*.

Although I tried to remind myself that these emotional side trips added time and delayed my efficiency, I often found myself taking them anyway. I was speechless when I came across the boxes that contained thousands of love poems. My father, the lyricist, had penned his poetry inside monthly "anniversary" cards he sent to his bride every month for six decades! The romance of that took my breath away. For a moment, I wondered if I were intruding. But even as part of me was wiping away my tears, the work-driven part was feeling inundated.

Too much stuff! I didn't want the responsibility for making all these decisions. Trying to figure out what to do with pounds and mounds of their memorabilia was complicated. One thing I discovered was unopened, unused items Lillian had collected over time—clothing, shoes, and even some expensive perfumes that had evaporated over time. I wondered what this collecting and stowing away was all about. I'm just the opposite, a woman who often wears new clothes directly out of the store, asking the sales clerk's help to detach the labels for me.

But like many of those young adults who survived the economic deprivations of the Great Depression after 1929, Mom was left with a condition some term "Depression mentality." These folks save things "just in case" they might need them someday. While cleaning out Dad's closet, I found that he, too, had amassed his own collections, although they were not of unused items. Dad's collection consisted of coins, stamps, record albums, and tapes.

What of all of this should I save and what do I throw away? How long should I keep the three copies of Mom's high school yearbook displaying Giggles's photo? Or even one of them? Who will ever want to look at them again? George Carlin was right: one person's treasure is another person's garbage. After we're gone, our treasures may seem worthless to our kids. And those love poems, should I even read them or were they too private? How many of the poems and cards should I keep? Five? Ten? Should I keep all of them? Would my parents ever ask for them again? Did they even know they had them now? And where would I put all this stuff?

I found the whole process very stressful, fraught with the chance that I might err big time. I feared my parents' future crestfallen faces: "Jane, you threw out my precious. . . ." These were hard decisions to make, harder still because it wasn't my stuff. I felt an odd sense of something that resembled betrayal when I let go of things that once seemed to have meant so much to my parents. Sometimes when I made these decisions about their stuff, they were resting in a nearby room. Most of the time they weren't present at all. On occasion I consulted Jack or Lillian about how I should deal with a certain item, but most of the time I just decided.

I sought to show my parents the appropriate deference and respect for their possessions. But my parents were never very materialistic people and, for all my concern of disappointing them or mis-categorizing their things, it turned out to be a nonissue with them. I recall having only one conversation about how I'd dealt with their possessions. It was with Dad and it occurred right after their move. Apparently, I questioned his wearing an olive-colored shirt. He responded that he was at a bit of a loss to know what to wear, since I'd thrown out or given away all of his favorite shirts. Nevertheless, he reassured me: "That's really okay with me, honey, they weren't that important. I guess this shade of green isn't my best color, huh?"

Despite my ordinary and very determined point of view that worrying is wasting precious energy, I so often found myself worrying during POP. And I "mis-worried" about so many events that never actually came about. Upsetting my parents by how I handled their stuff was apparently one of those. When it came down to it, my parents' stuff mattered relatively little to them. What really mattered to my parents was how I treated them.

THEIR STORY—MOM

It's strange how I felt as I watched my daughter go through all our boxes and total strangers pack up our belongings before our trip. I'd never liked having a lot of people in the apartment. That was why I let the plaster and paint remain like that for years and why it was so hard for me when the caregivers were here all the time.

In my younger days I might have been shocked to watch Jane read the love poetry Jack had written for me. Years ago, I might have taken offense having these moving men paw over my teenage photographs or our clothes. It might have felt like they were invading our privacy or that Jane was gaining access to my secrets, but today I find I don't mind they're being here in the same way.

At this point I can't recall all the things that I've collected over the course of my long life. There sure was a lot of it. When I was amassing the contents of all these boxes, what was inside them mattered to me—a lot. They represented pieces of my life. I cared a lot about what was inside these boxes, or, at least, I cared about the meaning I'd attached to them. But I've come to see many things differently since I piled these objects into the boxes. Today I care about the kindness Jane and her moving men have shown and the gentleness in how they treated me, Jack and our treasures.

Of course, I still value the wonderful cards and poetry my husband sent me each and every month on the 25th, our anniversary day. I'm also happy to have the letters Jane sent us from camp, school, or wherever she was. I kept lots of photos of our baby girl; she was so adorable. And I held on to the sweaters I'd knit for Jane and her dolls. I also had pictures of my parents and siblings from when we'd been young in those boxes. In the past, looking at some of those things had made me sad. But now, when Jane would come to us with Playbills from the Broadway shows we'd attended or the other memorabilia of times we'd had together, I was pleased to be reminded of things I had long forgotten.

I looked up and Jane was there, standing in a corner near the light, examining a shot of Jack and me when we first met. She was eyeing the photo carefully and I wondered what my daughter was seeing in it? I have a clear memory of that day, but I can't recall what I was like back then. Who was that young woman in the photo? I look so naive, so unsure of what I was to become or the life that would be ahead for the two of us. And Jack—his face is so unbelievably carefree and young! He's wearing those rimless spectacles that were so popular back in the 1940s. He looked handsome in them, so intelligent as he gazed at me with those kind eyes that won me over. I still love my husband's eyes and his intelligence. Can Jane see the love that was just starting that day between us? Is she imagining Jack and me before we'd even thought of having her?

As I look over all my things from the perspective of being an old woman, I feel detached from sadness or even nostalgia in a surprisingly good way. After years of working with psychotherapists, I've come to finally understand that I was really the one who'd attached any negative meaning to the events in my life. I probably cared too much that my things and I be "just right." My sensitivity to what others thought or said caused a lot of unnecessary pain. These days I'm trying to put a more uplifting meaning to my past. Jane says we can be calmer, Jack and I, if we focus less on our losses and more on savoring these moments we have together now and the good times we can recall. So, I'm trying that.

I'm even getting more relaxed about Jane's telling our story. If seeing the poems Jack wrote for me or reading about how we worked out things together as a family when Jack and I got older can help Jane help other people like us, where's the harm in that? I'm beginning to accept a lot of what's happening, maybe even our move to California.

YOUR STORY

Almost everyone has some emotional wounds left over from their childhood. You've already seen that my doing certain POP tasks, like packing up my childhood home or looking for an ALF, activated both remembrances and feelings that sometimes seemed "unreasonably" intense or even inexplicable. Perhaps that has happened to you as well. Despite sounding innocuous, dealing with your parents' stuff can be a minefield. It may surprise you how powerfully you react as you delve into your parents' belongings and memorabilia. You may unearth items you've never seen before and memories you may have long ago forgotten. Discovering childhood photos of you and your siblings or home movies of times when your parents were younger than you are now may "blow your mind."

Like me, you may spot a grainy photo of your Mom looking unrecognizably young and carefree, smiling up with wonder at her new "boyfriend," your Dad. He may be wearing a wide grin or a hairdo that was fashionable decades ago. You may stare at that shot for what seems like hours, imagining how your parents were when they first met or decided to have you.

When you've completed your POP tasks for the day and are available to fully listen to them, you'll learn a lot if you sit with your aging loved ones and invite them to tell you of their life joys or accomplishments. Since you and your parents may be sharing many feelings and memories, this time could prove a good one to strengthen your new POP relationship. You can mine your historic and loving connection by asking your parents to share their early memories. Even those parents with memory loss from dementia may recall their long-term memories. Do your best to be curious and have a nonjudgmental attitude. You will want to honor their stories or memories with compassion and perhaps a sweet appreciation for all they've been through in their lifetimes.

When you're examining the things that your parents saved over the course of their lives and talking with them in these ways, you may find that you're engaged in a kind of life review. That can elicit a variety of sentiments for all concerned. As a caring POParent you'll want to be sensitive in your responses, recognizing that sometimes a life review can result occasionally in your parents' emotional distress.

It's important to give yourself time and space to experience your own feelings during this "stuff-deciding" part of POP and other stages as well. Emotions like grief, nostalgia, regret, resentment, and others you didn't realize you had may come to the surface for you, too. Once they get triggered, you're likely to find it liberating to permit yourself to feel whatever comes up for you—be it the passage of time, your losses or the irony of parenting your own parents. In the moment, your feelings may challenge you; however, denying or avoiding your emotions and reactions eventually will inhibit the flow of your healing.

Even if you get sad or tear up, owning your feelings can connect you with your authentic self. You'll never want to shortchange giving yourself what you need to process what's been going on for you. Nonetheless, you can also decide to "delay reacting" until you're in the right place to take care of your own emotions. You may need to wait until you return to your home, partner, POP Family Coach, or friends to do so. Earlier you learned the value of underreacting while POParenting. Delayed reacting is another technique you will find useful, as it will help you regain a feeling of power over the things that *are* under your control—your own responses.

You may be sitting at your Mom's desk trying to make sense of her Medicare insurance premiums, and be surprised to find that you're having a lot of feelings. As your parents have gotten older, chances are they've acquired and kept a lot of papers. As attentive POParents you'll need to be discriminating as to what should be kept, filed, cleaned or tossed. Perhaps lately your parents have been less attentive about filing. You may encounter a lot of disorganized papers, bills, and other notices. You may also find yourself distressed at some of their recent decisions and want to undo some things your parents did late in life that they thought would be helpful—perhaps a reverse mortgage that isn't sound or a life insurance policy that makes little sense to you.

What your parents collected or chose to save reveals a great deal about them. Looking through their stuff may offer you a window into understanding them better and, in turn, help heal your relationship. Do their boxes contain your parents' finest memories or their darkest secrets? Have they turned into hoarders whose possessions have overtaken all available space and light in their house? Will they be offended by your disposing of their prized possessions?

As POParents, you and your siblings may well be deciding which of their things to keep and which to give away or even sell. If you're moving your parents to smaller quarters in a senior residence or in one of your homes, you can rent storage space for some of the things you or they can't stand to part with. You may discover that your wanting to hold on to their things is an unconscious way of holding on to your parents. There's nothing wrong with doing that, but you won't want to overdo it.

Parting with your parents' belongings can be really challenging. In general, we Americans like to keep our stuff. In 2010 the self-storage industry in the United States earned $20+ billion in annual revenues. I confess that I paid to keep some of my parents' things in storage after they moved to California and even after they had passed on.

You will also want to be attentive to the fact that packing up their home and looking over their "stuff" may stimulate irritability or even irrationality in your elderly parents, from your perspective. If they've already reached age eighty-five, like mine had a few years earlier, statistically one out of two of them will have some form of dementia, or cognitive impairment, including Alzheimer's. They will be least alert and least able to help you after the sun goes down (known clinically as "sun-downing"). They may demonstrate behaviors of people with dementia like "compensating," which may involve providing you answers when they don't know them and "perseverating," which is repeating themselves over and again.

It may disarm you when you first discover their long-term memories of events from the past are far sharper than their short-term memories—like what they ate for lunch. How else might these factors impact this part of your POP job? If you're pulling some golf trophy off the shelf and trying to decide if it stays or goes, you might ask your dad about its history. As he's recounting some long story, your mom may be grinning but not letting him see. She knows that those events never happened as he's telling it.

When they have certain diagnoses that affect their memories, your parents will do their best to remember, but when they can't recall a real answer, they may make one up. It's their way of dealing with not remembering at a certain stage of memory loss and shouldn't be seen by you as lying. Later in the course of their dementia, your aging loved ones won't recall and won't try to pretend they do. Later still, they won't try to recall and you won't ask them to. Understanding their conditions and where they are progressively, if your parents' diseases are progressive, will help you make better POP decisions as well as be less perturbed by their seemingly quirky behaviors.

Similarly, with "perseverating," if your parents repeat themselves, ask you the same question over and again in the same conversation or call you with the same query several times in the same hour, it can try your patience. They're unaware they're perseverating. Even if you've heard the story about your dad's golf trophy often in the past, when you bring it down from the shelf, you may choose to patiently hear it again. And you may hear it again a short time later if your father asks, "Honey, did I ever tell you about the time I won that golf trophy?" Employing the compassion and patience you've been cultivating will help you deal with these moments.

Even if your parents don't have a form of dementia or debilitating disorder, your poking around in their things may be frustrating or upsetting to them and they may not be happy with the whole idea. Your parents' reactions may even be inconsistent from one day to the next. Like your children, they may react differently to your good ideas from one sleepy night to the next rested morning. Or on Saturday your parents may seem grateful for your help in packing them up but on Sunday, they may have become upset or confused at what you've done with their things. If you are in a hurry with this part of your POP tasks, you may prefer to not ask them for much help or to do this when your folks are out of their house or sleeping.

Certainly, your parents are likely to have many feelings about parting with their home and the possessions they spent a lifetime amassing—some of these feelings may be both positive and negative. For example, your folks may like having fewer things to be responsible for and may appreciate your downsizing or de-cluttering but still resent what may seem like your "intrusiveness." Resisting giving away certain things—like their 45 RPM records with no turntable to play them on—may be your parents' way of holding on to their memories or of retaining some control to offset feeling overwhelmed and full of grief.

Even if your parents' possessions seem old, out of date, or unattractive to you, they may turn out to provide great comfort or joy to them. Those 45s may turn into an unexpected gold mine on eBay and provide them a great way to share their memories with young people who are interested buyers. Just as your daughter's beloved blanket was such a consolation that she refused to let you wash it, your mom's silk pillowcases may be a treasure you shouldn't mess with. Some of you have parents of my generation who still carry around the fearful "Depression mentality" from 1929 or from the stock market crash in 2008, and they may be reluctant to let any stuff go, no matter how much they have. That will make this POP job all the tougher for you.

You might be able to turn some of your POP sorting and organizing into donations for needy individuals and charitable entities. Giving things to others less fortunate can feel good for your parents and you. Plus, those deductible donations may also help them when tax time rolls around. Well-planned and advertised garage sales could yield some money for things you and they don't want to transport. Craigslist, eBay, and many online sites offer opportunities to turn your parents' items into cash for them. Selling your parents' coin collections, vintage clothing, and vinyl records can become a source of unexpected income. Your parents are likely to be grateful for any increase to their finances and proud of you for demonstrating your ingenuity to see money where they did not.

The division of your parents' stuff can pose a serious hazard for siblings who are co-POParenting. Don't be surprised to find yourselves disagreeing with your siblings, sometimes over emotional reactions and sometimes over the stuff itself. Since family members have a stake in the outcome, they're likely to have their own ideas of how and what to do with your parents' keepsakes, vintage items, and their stock portfolio, too. Various siblings will want some things and some of you will want the same things. Some may think items should be sold and others will have different opinions. This is where I like to point out the advantages of being an only child: you get to take all the stuff you want and nobody argues with you about it.

When you have siblings, however, everything is a bit different and may require delicate negotiating. All of you may want to own the special tea set your dad brought back from Japan after World War II, but only one of you will end up winning that round. On the other hand, there would be no negotiating if you see the torn ticket stub from your parents' first date as trash while your sister sees it as a nostalgic treasure she wants to keep. Over the years, your parents may have promised to leave some of their things to you or to various siblings. Those bequests may now create unpleasant friction within your family, a family who is also operating as TEAM POP.

Consider how you and your family can avoid the foreseeable risks of family discord. Talk with each other candidly and kindly. Utilize today's technology like Skype and FaceTime to set up family meetings, not just to deal with POP issues but to share yourselves with your distant siblings on holidays. If you think your family could benefit from some help, try some POP Family Coaching or other family counseling with a pastoral or counseling professional. The seeds of future controversy, quarreling, and even litigation, can be removed before they take root at this stage of your POPcycle. When your parents have left the planet, your siblings will hopefully be a source of continued love and devotion; it's important to pay attention to your family's well-being and not expect the healing and good feelings to automatically occur without your paying them some focused attention.

Another good way to avoid such potential infighting is to discern when unfinished emotional business is taking the place of rational discourse and choices. That is, notice carefully if you and/ or your siblings are bringing unrelated matters into your conversations about what to do with your parents' possessions. That may hypothetically take many forms. One may include such catty remarks as: "Sure, you want Mom's mink coat. You always liked those luxury items Mom had. But why do *you* need her coat? You found a husband who buys you lots of them. It's just like when we were kids, you thought you were entitled to all Mom's pretty stuff that she didn't use anymore. You remember the pink taffeta dress . . ." and so on.

Family relations will improve if each of you separates out the past issues from the present time. Everyone needs to stay on task in POP, as intrafamily squabbling over inequities or antiquities from the past will only serve to undermine your best efforts. Talk about how to make wise decisions together today and focus on your parents' best interests. What's wanted and needed today among POParent-siblings is family unity. Avoid making comments that interpret people's behavior rather than resolve the issues. Stay away from trying to prove something about the past with your siblings. Don't attribute a meaning to which sibling gets what possessions from your parents' estate or who is allowed to do what with your parents' things; doing so can easily divert your collective attention away from the main thrust of POP.

My advice is to do all you can to avoid seeding more family problems into your future. Since your siblings will predictably be here long after your parents are no longer around, aim to be considerate to their sensitivities even as you're learning to be a more loving POParent. Every family has its strengths and limitations. Greed, bitterly spoken differences of opinion, sarcasm, and disdainful judgments can undermine or even destroy the very harmony you're trying to construct.

It might be that you're arguing because you're really just sad that your folks will eventually leave the planet and abandon you. It might be human nature to argue about stuff if the anger is easier to tolerate than the sadness. We need to face the fact that some people in every family are more concerned with money and material things than others. It's likely they've been acting that way for decades. If that conduct reappears now in this setting, and it's likely it will, staying on target with your POP mission will help you to weaken its divisive impact on your family: after all, POP's not about the money; it's about your folks.

10

SETTLING OUR PARENTS INTO THEIR NEW LIVES

MY STORY

I have always been fascinated with how the human brain works. So, after bringing my parents out to California, I wondered why they, as smart as they were, tolerated so many numbing East Coast winters when they could have long ago come out to live in the sunshine—where their joints wouldn't ache from the cold and their only child could come by for lunch? Had they seen themselves as pioneers from New Jersey or survivors of challenges? Maybe the way Frank Sinatra had crooned of New Yorkers: "if I can make it there, I'll make it anywhere."[1]

But years of practicing psychotherapy had taught me that people have different values and, therefore, their reasoning can seem a bit inexplicable to others with different priorities. I'd also learned that my road to greater contentment lay in being grateful that my parents were here now, rather than understanding why it had taken so long to get them here. There were innumerable things I wanted to do so my folks would feel welcome.

Now that I'd started making many of their important decisions, my main goal was to help them enjoy healthier, richer lives in their California setting. While doing POP long distance, my default position had been to be overly protective. In the past, I'd erred on the side of doing more than was necessary for them rather than less. I'd thought long and hard and always planned ahead. I had lots of Plan B's, C's, and even a few D's. I was the POPoster Mom for "Be prepared!" Maybe that had been my way of compensating for not being in the same city where they lived. But now that I was virtually "down the block," I wanted to get it right and avoid doing so much for them that I might undermine their sense of independence and self-confidence, I had seen other POParents "over-do" their attention and involvement. I would need to discover the right balance—and, as they aged and we continued the POPcycle, I knew that right balance point would move.

How would I know when to help? How could I accurately hit the mark and do neither too much nor too little for them? The last thing I wanted was to undermine my parents' dignity or negate their skills. Particularly when they were first getting used to their assisted-living facility (ALF) and to our new relationship in this California location, I wanted Mom to feel comfortable that I wasn't going to micromanage everything or run her life. I wanted Dad to know that my "helping" would fall far short of cutting his food into little cubes.

My goal was to see what worked for Lillian and Jack in their ALF and then do more of that. I figured that the three of us would do our best if I stood back a bit and took a little time to observe how they were doing on their own at the ALF. Breathing through my angst about not having everything figured out immediately, I reminded myself that such a thing was impossible, as things just took longer with aging parents. But it was wonderful to realize that I too could slow down! I just needed to better observe how they were faring in their new environment.

When I slowed down and held the intention to observe rather than assume that I knew what would be best for them, I was better able to discover what was actually occurring. Thus, I also learned to be more discerning. I found I could more clearly hear when my parents needed me and when they didn't. Maybe I could even wait until they asked for my help. I wanted them to feel confident and to keep "stretching," and now I wondered again: If I didn't run in so quickly, would they and could they do more for themselves?

Since beginning POP, I'd always encouraged Mom and Dad to be as self-sufficient as possible. I knew that by being too protective, whatever that was, I might be undermining their ability to do things for themselves. That situation could also make them lazy and become depressing to them, weakening the very "muscles" we all wanted strengthened.

Finding that fine line between too much and not enough help, and then living up to it, was challenging because it was ever changing. In spite of starting many a visit promising myself to do no more than was warranted, I often found myself drifting into "autopilot," as I now termed it, and "over-parenting" them. I'd be lifting something they could easily move or offering to make a dinner arrangement when they were perfectly capable of doing that for themselves. When I saw it, I'd stop myself. I could see I was beginning to treat my own parents like they were children, not the adults with some limitations they truly were. I knew that my continuing to act in that way wouldn't be good for our relationship. So, in addition to subtly watching them, I kept a watch on myself as well.

Aiming to make their transition seamless, I reviewed what they had needed Florence to do. When Jack and Lillian had still been in their NYC home, they'd needed minimal physical help from Florence on the five days each week she was there. She assisted with a few of their basic activities of daily living (ADLs) like taking baths and dressing. But most of her work had involved assisting them with their instrumental activities of daily living (IADLs), like seeing that they took their medications; food shopping, preparation, and cleanup; housecleaning; and laundry. Florence also had accompanied and transported Mom and Dad to their doctor appointments, rehab, haircuts, and trips to the accountant at tax season.

Many of those tasks would now be done for my parents by me or at the ALF. Their bathrooms would be cleaned, healthy meals prepared, and other domestic matters attended to. Mom and Dad would also be furnished a variety of new recreational and health opportunities such as exercise programs, outings, lectures, and trips to the mall. I'd anticipated having to pay for a fair number of extra hours of caregiving once they were at the ALF and was pleasantly surprised to learn how little additional help they seemed to need.

Before long, Mom and Dad were participating in their new life and community. The ALF had its own rhythm and schedules, and they seemed to have no trouble adapting to it. They were happily taking the van to the mall to do some small shopping trips and remarking on how good the food tasted. Mom was even attending some chair yoga classes.

Now that they were finally close by, I looked forward to more direct contact with their medical providers. I went about the process of interviewing and hiring a small medical team for them and then watched it grow. They needed a dentist, cardiologist, eye doctor, audiologist, geriatric internist, and geriatric psychiatrist. I also wanted my parents to go to my longevity specialist, hoping that seeing him would lengthen and strengthen their lifetime with me. Eventually, they both would also have to undergo the cataract surgeries that almost all older parents have, requiring another specialist. Dad's fall would need us to have a brain surgeon and a whole rehab team; Mom's fall would require an orthopedic surgeon and several rehab teams as well. But I get ahead of myself.

I was recommended to a kind dentist who had retirement in his future in a nearby town and set up an initial appointment there for Lillian and Jack. I researched a good local optometrist and arranged for them to get new glasses. Repeatedly, I took a frustrated Mom to her very patient audiologist. Improving the quality of hearing can be an almost impossible goal, as I have discovered, even with my very wealthy older patients who could pay anything for better hearing aids, but Mom's audiologist tried over and again.

I trekked with my aging parents the hour and a half drive each way to work with Dr. Barry Fox, the well-respected "longevity doctor" I used. Getting Mom and Dad to make the long ride into downtown Los Angeles to see him was tough. But I insisted. A contemporary of my folks, Barry was still actively practicing medicine and dispensing sage advice, dietary supplements after testing for their body's deficits, and other disease prevention measures. Barry was always inspiring, and I wanted my parents to receive the same high-quality holistic care I sought for myself.

By taking them to these doctor visits, I got to know their physicians fairly well. Most of them were immensely kind and caring to my mother and father, but I also knew that older patients receive more thorough medical attention when a POParent attends the visit with them. I considered my POP job to extend far beyond being the driver. I actively participated, asked probing questions my parents didn't think to ask or felt intimidated about because doctors are authority figures. I also helped by gently correcting my parents' short-term recall of recent events or even their long-term memory. After the visits, I would follow up with them to see they were adhering to their doctor's requirements and reminding them of the subtler suggestions they hadn't heard or remembered to do.

Back in the day when it was less common to do so, many of my parents' physicians gave me access to them beyond ordinary office hours via their cell phones. I was delighted to be able to locate such competent and generous people. I knew, from some of those POP families I'd personally coached, that this wasn't a usual practice at that time, but my family and I were very fortunate in this regard too, and I will always be very grateful.

By now it was becoming natural for me to take care of things for them all the time—to be the parent—instead of the other way around, as it used to be. My next step, after seeking to advance their health, was helping with their finances. I set up a meeting at a neighborhood bank branch, introduced them to their new banker, and opened a checking account for them. I arranged for their Social Security checks to be deposited directly into their new account, so they'd have their money regularly deposited without any effort on their part. I was listed as a cosignatory on their checking account, so I could write checks for them and, should there be a problem, I would be advised. Since I ended up writing all their checks—for caregiver care, medicine, and supplemental insurance—and balanced their accounts, they never met the banker again.

I also took on as my POP job to arrange for much of my parents' cultural lives when they were newly in town. I modeled myself on the way I'd seen them raise me in this regard and felt like I was somehow honoring them when I followed their lead in my POParenting. I was very young when my parents first introduced me to music, comedy, and art, sharing their love of these with me. Even when they could barely afford the price of admission, Jack and Lillian felt it important to expose their young daughter to theater, museums, and even opera, which they didn't particularly like.

I was actually seven when my parents took me to my first Broadway play, *Inherit the Wind*. It was an amazing spectacle with brilliant acting, writing, and directing. The play reenacted the famous Scopes trial from the 1920s when a Southern teacher is banned from teaching the truth of evolution to his students. Seeing on stage how lawyers could play such a meaningful role in bringing about or blocking societal change and being incredibly moved by all I saw, I decided—then and there—to become an attorney so I, too, could do good.

Now it was my turn to take Jack and Lillian to plays, art museums, and cultural events in twenty-first-century Los Angeles. What a surprise I had in store for me! Far more important than the entertainment being presented to my folks was their own level of physical comfort. They no longer enjoyed walking around museums or being driven through them in wheelchairs. The effort it took them to get to and exit from the theater, their difficulty hearing the performers, and their dislike of "missing dinner" at the ALF began to be insurmountable barriers to the cultural enrichment I was trying to provide them. What a lesson! Part of me wanted my parents to want to go to cultural events but if I really listened to what they wanted, they wanted to stay home most of the time. I began to wonder for whom was I offering these opportunities. Them? Or me so I could still see them as more vibrant and into living as they had been when they were younger?

So, I realized I would have to adapt. I tried coming up with fun opportunities that might be more comfortable for my aging parents. My motivation was good: I didn't want their worlds to become any smaller. I wanted to keep their brains engaged and to heed the warning of "use it or lose it." But this, like many other things, wasn't up to me.

After a while, I learned from them. As a result, Mom, Dad, and I spent many an afternoon visiting around the radio, like the days of their youth before television. I found the local "time of your life" radio stations that played old show tunes and even some standards that Jack himself had written. We'd sing along.

I watched my father relish his peaceful times. He'd borrow a book from the residents' library, settle into a comfortable chair, take off his glasses and be in heaven. I'd smile finding him buried under his book. When Dad's memory started to fail him, I'd sometimes notice he was reading the same book more than once. It reminded me of children endlessly craving their favorite book or DVD. Rereading never seemed to bother the very young or the very old. I tried to not let it bother me either.

Decades earlier, doing the Sunday *New York Times* crossword puzzles was a family ritual we'd all engaged in and loved. Lillian had been the real puzzle champion, completing the *Times* puzzles daily—and in pen, a real feat. Especially after her diagnosis of Alzheimer's, the fact that she continued to try her hand at them so delighted me that I made a deal with her: for the rest of her days, as long as she wanted new puzzle books, I'd happily buy them.

Next, I checked out their new neighborhood's religious opportunities, something they'd done for me so long ago. Their ALF had religious people who held services there on special holidays and other occasions. Even though my parents weren't very involved in their religion, the fact that their ALF offered a piece of their own cultural tradition right there at home helped to make their transition easier.

Mom and Dad liked dining at the ALF and the regularity of the meals and menu offerings there. Nonetheless, they also enjoyed my taking them out to eat, and doing so became one of our new rituals, especially after they lost interest in going to plays or concerts. They were particularly snooty about their New York delicatessens. "Jane, you're out in the West. None of these delis can touch the Madison Deli near the apartment or the Stage in midtown," they'd boast with personal pride. Of course, they were right. They knew their New York fare.

On holidays, I'd try to take them out somewhere special. My requirements for such restaurants during our POPcycle were: they'd tried it before and already liked it, the acoustics permitted carrying on a conversation, it was located a short drive from their ALF, and it had a patient wait staff.

My Mom had been a foodie and used to share her joy of trying new tastes with me. However, at this juncture, her taste buds and sense of smell were, as most of us in our late eighties, dulled by age and maybe a bit by eating the food at the ALF three times a day. So, like with kids, my mother would often celebrate holidays by eating too much of a new taste or gorging on a large meal and then a gooey dessert. Getting her home before she got sick in the car was itself a challenge. I had forgotten that reality until writing this, which makes me see how, as so often happens with POParenting, I've filtered my memories through the mist of time passing and missing my parents.

Neither Jack nor Lillian seemed to be making new friends easily, if at all, at the ALF. Dad was content reading, watching his shows on television, and spending his time with Mom and with me. He didn't find any men who really interested him as friends, and I could understand how his unusual profession and life experiences might make it hard to find peers. One day I approached him and talked about his absence of sociability, to which he replied: "Look around, Jane. Think about my interests and the life I've had. I just don't see anyone here I'd really want to spend much time with, aside from you and your Mom, of course. Would you want to be friends with these guys?"

I thought about trying to fix this problem. I even went so far as to check out the more sophisticated-looking couples at their AL when I visited. But I drew the line at setting up playdates for my parents. Talk about overprotecting them!

As Mom and Dad were becoming somewhat familiar faces at their new home, I did come up with one idea that had some socializing overtones. The ALF often staged theme-centered evenings for the residents and, when I approached the administrator with the idea of holding an event—a Frank Sinatra evening with live singing—she was game. The evening turned out to be a huge success. The social director/singer crooned out all the favorite Sinatra songs, including a few written by Dad. Jack didn't say a whole lot about it, but he looked really pleased. As I'd hoped, this garnered him some brief celebrity status at the facility, and Mom and I had a blast, too.

As I was figuring out how to become a better local POParent, I aimed to include some of the POP Family Coaching tools I'd recommended that had proven useful to other families. One such technique involves approaching your own parents as if they were complete strangers. When we meet new people, even on airplanes, we often relate to them with curiosity and much interest rather than assuming we already understand them or their motivations. What I hoped to do with that tool was to develop the ability to experience these people I already know well as if they were new to me, to hear what they're saying with a kind of neutral fascination.

I wanted to try that out and act as if these intimates of mine were new to me. In a way, my parents were new people to me. We'd been living apart for over thirty-five years, and each of us had grown and experienced so much during that time. If I could give up the idea (for this exercise) that I knew them well, or was supposed to, I might actually be able to "meet" my parents where they were now.

When I became able to offer Jack and Lillian the respect, inquiry, and interest I gave to new people, my relationship with them improved dramatically. It wasn't that hard to do, since I truly aimed to discover who Lillian and Jack had become as people over these decades, aside from simply being my parents. This required that I ask more questions, listen more fully to their responses, and pass fewer judgments. By making just these slight alterations, I noticed my parents began to feel more respected and more at ease with their move, as did I.

Another technique I teach others in POP Family Coaching that I thought would be useful to apply at this time was "reframing." I have spoken previously with you about this well-respected tool. I teach family members how to look more neutrally, without so much emotion, at what's actually occurring in order to discover other ways to interpret what's happening by thinking differently. This allows us to take a pause and not react automatically or overly emotionally. By using our intelligence to assign a more uplifting interpretation to events, we can change our moods and expand our options for solutions. When I pictured the scenario of my parents' move as dragging my enfeebled elderly parents to their last resting place in a senior institution, I felt horrible. But when I reframed what was happening, I could see the situation as welcoming dear old friends/parents to their new home, town, and new life. Thinking about it this way, I felt less depressed. It wasn't that I was fooling myself; rather I was adding another, different point of view into my thinking that resulted in my feeling calmer and, actually, better able to help them.

Settling my folks into their new life in California—finding them their ALF, doctors, banker, and delicatessen—was yet another opportunity to see the "role reversal," or the "Circle of Life," as some of us prefer to call it. I favor the term "Circle of Life" to explain my POP experience because it evokes a sense of continuity, predictability, and unending connection. The term "role reversal," may be challenging if it suggests interfering with the natural order and that things are somehow being forced backward in the universe. Taking care of an aging Lillian and Jack felt oddly right to me, even orderly.

I had the thought that I really wanted to become a better POParent to them than my parents had been to me. I wasn't coming from the position of being competitive, but I wanted to become the best me—whether I was being a POParent, a lawyer, or a therapist. I loved it when I could exceed my own previous levels of POParental patience or kindness. I felt like I was healing spots in my own heart when I could act even more compassionately when parenting them than they had when parenting me. Jack and Lillian weren't the only ones changing. I was changing too.

The direction of the POPcycle is relentless: my parents did become more and more dependent, and I became more and more responsible. Once I'd begun managing certain things for my folks, they never asked to regain control of those things. Our roles and functions were in constant flux, going one way, and that required dexterity on my part. The only reliable POP predictor was unpredictability, but, at least now, I had my parents settled in and closer to me. A long-distance phone call wouldn't be all I had to help me diagnose a stroke or prevent a suicide. I could be right there.

THEIR STORY—MY MOTHER-IN-LAW, EVAN

When my beloved husband Al died in the late 1970s, I suffered an amazing loss in my life. Fortunately, our sons were incredibly supportive and my career as a high-powered magazine editor was still in high gear back then. My children, who lived all over the country, encouraged me to continue my life, even marry another man two years later. And so I did.

My second husband was an advertising executive that Al and I had known in business for over twenty years. We too had a fine marriage, but after fourteen years, it was cut short when he died in Houston where we'd moved. Dealing with my second widowhood, I returned to New York City shortly thereafter and retired unofficially. I was seventy-nine then.

I traveled to Europe and Asia with women friends whom I had cherished all my life and for a while, that was fascinating. But inevitably, age took its toll and travel became more complicated. Eventually even the pleasure of visiting my two older sons where they lived, far from New York was undermined because of how exhausting the travel had become for me.

Soon thereafter, I also took several falls. One of those required my temporarily living in a home to recuperate fully. My three sons apparently talked together and reached a consensus: because I already needed some help at my own place and because of my advanced age, their mom would need to leave the elegant apartment she cherished. She could either move into a secure senior citizen facility—one that would accommodate her and her priceless architecturally designed modern furniture, paintings, and sculpture—or she could move in with one of them.

Live with my children? *No way!* I adore them and their families, but living with them in their homes would be trouble and trauma! But could I live in a senior facility full of old folks whom I believed would be standoffish or suspicious of a newcomer or some hot shot "career lady?" *No way!* Where did those two "options leave me now, I wondered?

The kids persisted, pressing me for a final decision. As I now like to say, I chose the lesser of two evils. While "screaming and kicking," I opted for a senior facility where I could live in my own apartment with my own things and could eat as many meals as I wished to pay for. In the new facility I could swim, watch movies, and invite my boys and their families to the private dining room for holiday dinners with me. The staff here knows to call up to my apartment if I don't show up somewhere in the building by 10:30 in the morning. I am independent *and* my sons feel safe!

To act like the editor I once used to be—and make this long wonderful story shorter—within a month of arriving there, I was asked to manage our facility's library. That job is something I've done and adore doing all these years later. Most importantly within six months of my arrival, I'd met six new women who were the most wonderful people, right here in my own building. They've become my dear friends, museum companions, and loving confidantes.

Had I not gone along when my kids insisted on it, I might not have come here or to a place like this until much later in my life if at all. Had I put off facing the inevitable—I wouldn't always be able to care for myself—I feel certain that the best part of my years here, the companionship piece, might never have occurred. Part of the beauty of my sons' timing was that I was still able to make new and deep connections with other people. I've seen with other new residents that if they arrive here too late in their lives, it can be really difficult to make new friends and have a good time with other peers.

Now when my family comes to visit, they kid me that I can't find the time in my busy agenda to see them. Well, that's not really true and never will be. I'll always make time for them. I speak my mind and do so loudly, and I love my sons most for not allowing my possible displeasure to stop them from saying and doing what they knew was right for me.

I see that my children have indeed become my parents, and I toast them and their POParenting ways. They must have had a good role model!

YOUR STORY

Moving is stressful at any age. If you're taking your older parents away from the comforts of their home, the places they're familiar with and things they know, you can plan on having some stressful days. You will need to manage your own as well as your parents' anticipated angst. You will also need to respond to their questions, however many times they may ask. You may find yourself absorbing a lot of emotions. And, if your parents are like mine, they will worry before the move, as it's happening, and maybe even after it's over. But sooner or later, they will begin to enjoy their new life. And after a while, hopefully, they'll be grateful to you for where they've landed.

If your parents can comprehend it, your first step will be to explain the whole move to them from start to finish. In many ways, their understanding the scenario is less important than their confidence that you know what you're doing. It's likely they'll want to know at least the following: when is the move; how will it happen; who will help; what will happen to their valuables; how will the furniture from their three-story house fit into a one-bedroom unit.

Do not underestimate the significance of your parents' leaving their home—their place of dominion and control—forever. Even if your parents aren't very talkative and even if it feels odd, it will help if you invite them to sit down and share all their concerns about the move with you, one-by-one. Listen fully. Respond kindly and be as specific in your answers as is appropriate to their level of understanding. Never make fun of any of your parents' worries. You may want to dismiss your folks as classic worriers or believe that what they're bothered by isn't very important.

I learned over time to take my parents' expressed concerns seriously. Even many years after Mom was diagnosed with dementia, any time she expressed a complaint, I found that I needed to carefully check it out. You should honor and respectfully evaluate your parents' apprehensions and complaints.

Their upcoming move may be one where your parents are in less control than at any other time in their adult lives. Under the stress, they may become aggressive because of their current lack of control or their inability to remember information you've already told them. For your dad who will no longer be able to putter around in the garage or have his special room to watch the games in, leaving home can be depressing. Your parents may be sad at losing the companionship of dear friends or the delights of their old neighborhood. Your mom may say it wasn't in her plans to lose her kitchen, her sewing room, or her tub. She too may leave home kicking and screaming, like Evan, or worse yet, bawling like a child.

Think of what this move must be like for your parents or your beloved in-laws, who may by now have a limited sense of hearing, sight, and smell, and may have limited funds as well. They're watching brawny strangers handling their precious, breakable possessions and packing up their undergarments. They're leaving almost everyone they know to go to a place they've never even seen near "their daughter-in-law's house." They can't take all their furniture and beloved art with them because they're going into a small apartment or your house. They're afraid of losing lifelong neighborhood friends and that no one will call them long distance on their new phone number (which they're having trouble remembering). And they're departing from the home where they raised you, maybe recovered from cancer, maybe grieved the death of your sister, faced whatever events of their life story that took place within those walls.

Your ability to demonstrate your POP compassion at this significant moment may make a big difference to your relationship with your mom and dad. Aim to keep engaging with your parents and attending to their requests with patience even when they repeat themselves. This will help keep them grounded and will add to their confidence in you. During the move, your focus will need to be on resolving logistics and on your parents' immediate concerns.

The move may itself bring up some latent fears your parents have been having, as it is full of potential trauma. At some later point, after they're settled in, depending on your parents' capabilities to do so, you may wish to address deeper, underlying fears they may be contemplating or even obsessing over, such as their own mortality or concerns about your or your siblings' future. By being in an ongoing dialogue with them, hopefully you can allay some of these worries or bring them to a professional who can help.

Days before the move, you will have asked your parents to select (or you can choose for them, if they can't) some of their treasured items to hand-carry to their new home. These things will likely evoke welcoming feelings for them in the new place. Consistency is very calming. Seeing and touching their familiar, loved things in their new residence may mitigate some of the negative feelings your parents have associated with leaving home. The more infirm your parents have become, the more they may enjoy having a few of their favorite objects around when they arrive.

If you can bring familiar smells, tastes, and sights in their new place, that could ease some of the challenge to your parents' transition. Doing this may be easiest when your parents are moving into your home (or that of one of your siblings) where cooking traditional foods, perhaps using your mom's recipes, is common, or other traditions reminiscent of their cultural roots are present. Your decision to lug your dad's favorite TV chair and ottoman to his new home, heavy though they were, may make all the difference in his feeling comfortable there. And if you're moving your parents to this country from overseas, bring along some of their favorite regional foods and find a place to refresh your supply: that alone could prove more valuable than you can imagine.

Your kids likely trained you as parents to bring along a beloved stuffed animal, however ragged, wherever you took them. I recommend you apply a similar principle if your parents have to spend time in a lonely hospital room. Bring along one or two of your parent's favorite objects. Handling those things may lower your parent's blood pressure and speed recovery. Seeing the beloved treasure or trinket can trigger a feeling of being loved and safe.

Once your parents have arrived at their new home, you can take a series of deep breaths. The first thing you'll want to do is lower your expectations of your parents' immediate appreciation and joy. They may react much less positively than you'd hoped. Even if you're certain their new home is safer, cleaner, and now closer to you, don't expect them to share your view that it's necessarily better. Not yet. Give your parents some time to adjust (remember "old dogs and new tricks"). Remember that you carefully chose their new place and that major adjustments take some time to absorb.

This is the time to consider how else to make your parents feel settled. If your mom loves playing canasta, maybe you can find her a game where she's at a similar skill level with her fellow players. If your dad would still like to putter with tools but doesn't have his garage to do so anymore, maybe you can enroll him in a shop class or ask him to do a small work task at your home.

If your parents are too aged to socialize much or aren't very talkative, you might consider getting them a pet—presuming it's allowed in their new facility. The permission to bring pets may play a role in your decision of which facility best suits your parents. Being around domesticated animals can provide extraordinary companionship and make a real difference in the quality of your parents' lives. Just be wary about any type or breed that might require too much maintenance.

Since many seniors have limited intimate physical contact and get touched only occasionally, they can suffer from a kind of failure to thrive like an infant when left untouched. Who knows, maybe a cat or a bird could provide your parents a whole new lease on life. I've seen it happen. Because of the therapeutic benefits, there are agencies that bring trained animals to visit in nursing homes. If your parents' facility doesn't already do so, you might ask them to consider it.

For their own protection, there may come a time, and usually does in every POPcycle when you (or someone on TEAM POP) will need to take over some or all of the financial and legal aspects of your folks' life—their checkbooks, investments, dealings with Medicare, and so on. How will you know when that is? Your parents' geriatrician may advise you, or your parents may give you clues that your involvement is appropriate. You may discover they've paid someone twice, having forgotten that they'd already sent a check. Older parents are frequent victims of financial fraud schemes, so you will want to be alert to take on their finances before something dire occurs.

It may be that a small step is all that's needed. Helping your parents with their money often involves small incremental changes, like much of POP. You may go from no information to being emailed copies of your parents' bank account statements on a monthly basis to being added to the accounts as a cosignatory.

Even more serious steps may become appropriate in your family. Taking the proper steps in a timely fashion may help shield your parents from real disaster. Based upon your continuing observations of your parents' abilities and shortcomings, the designated person may now be writing all their checks and making all their fiscal and investment decisions. Wherever your parents are on this part of the POPcycle, when you're moving them to a new location, that's often a very good time to make some needed changes.

Taking over many financial responsibilities relieved my parents and me of much anxiety. Although some elderly parents will be relieved, others may be of two minds about your having this type, or extent, of control over their affairs. Your parents may resist, especially if you approach it right after their move. At that moment, although your mom and dad will appreciate having you there to back them up, they may feel they've lost so much control—over their homes, bodily functions, and even their minds—that they'll hesitate to cede more control, especially over their finances. Should this be an issue, you or the banker, broker, or accountant should patiently explain to your parents the benefits of having a second person on their account to review their statements, balance their accounts, and deal with any delinquency notices.

You will want to scout out your folks' new locale for whatever else they need or want nearby. For your family, that may mean golf courses, churches, shoe repair stores, vegan restaurants, or yoga studios. Before signing them up with a pharmacy, you'll want to know if it is on your parents' Medicare Plan, delivers prescriptions, is open 24/7, offers flu shots, and crosschecks your parents' medications for dangerous drug interactions. Like me, you'll want to help your parents find physicians, caregivers, and maybe even new friends. You may have to sign them up for phone, internet, or other communication services and then show them, over and over, how to use the remote control or the default settings.

Finally, as you aim to bring your parents into the twenty-first century, you may wish to share with them some of the advantages and advances in alternative and complementary medicines. Today many doctors trained in Western medicine agree that there are numerous positive results achieved with practices that might have been considered unorthodox or untested in your parents' youth. Similarly, many reputable studies have validated a number of techniques that at one time seemed more questionable.

Your parents may find their painful and chronic conditions vastly improved by practices such as yoga, meditation, acupuncture and acupressure, chiropractic adjustments, or visualization techniques. Medicare may not yet pay for some practices and procedures, such as use of appropriate supplements for aging bodies, naturopathic substances instead of pharmaceuticals, and other alternative treatments, but things are changing. You may need to advocate for anything outside of the ordinary with your parents' providers and convince your parents of the value for them of anything outside their comfort zone. But as good POParents, one of the things you can try to do is to get your aging loved ones better health in their new homes.

Sooner or later, the time will come when your whirlwind of tasks begins to quiet down; your parents will find themselves adjusting to their move, and you will adapt too. Maybe you'll even hear them say they're enjoying their new home and transplanted lives.

11

TRYING TO MAKE A PERMANENT POPLAN

Do You Want to See God Laugh?

MY STORY

One evening I picked up my folks to take them out to dinner. I'd last seen them only a couple of days earlier and we'd talked on the phone daily since then. Dad had been lucid and I'd not been alerted to any problems. We had an evening of good food and laughter, but afterward, I was troubled by the slowness of Dad's gait as he walked from our table to the door of the restaurant. Although he was moving at the speed of molasses, my father seemed unaware of anything amiss. When we got to the car, I watched as he slowly and deliberately inched his way onto the seat.

I asked him specific questions about any recent events that might have triggered this particular change. He demurred and seemed confused. I wasn't sure how reliable his memory might be, so I continued inquiring until he volunteered, "Maybe this has something to do with the fall I took in our bathroom a while back."

"What fall? You took a fall in the bathroom? How long ago? How come this is the first I'm hearing of it?" I sputtered out, trying to ask four questions at once and sound patient all at the same time. "You know. When I fell and hit my head the other day," he answered.

Apparently, Jack had slipped and fallen in their bathroom and then "neglected" to mention it to me or to anyone else on the assisted-living facility (ALF) staff. It looked like Dad's fall had occurred nearly a month before! Upon questioning, he recalled hitting his head on the way down as he tried unsuccessfully to break his fall. He said he'd told Mom right after he'd pulled himself up from the floor in the bathroom. Likely she'd forgotten about the event soon thereafter. Generally speaking, she was no longer a reliable person to prompt Dad to remember things, since she didn't recall that much herself.

I tried to underreact—that technique described earlier that has worked for me repeatedly. I didn't want to chide my father, like he was a bad child for not informing a more appropriate person about his fall and head injury, someone with a better memory, than Mom. But I would have appreciated not having to wait a month to hear about and then respond to the potential repercussions of this fall. My being able to react quickly to things like the fall he'd taken was a big part of why I'd brought my parents closer in the first place. Hadn't I planned on being able to keep more current with their lives here?

What happened to that portion of our POPlan? Now, even with my parents living closer, I still felt out of the information loop. I was beginning to see that neither the short distance between their home and mine nor the small amount of time between visits would ensure I'd always be timely informed about everything POP. What were the implications of that, I wondered?

In the morning I arranged for the earliest possible visit with Dad's geriatric physician, since I recognized that a blow to the head of an elderly man could be highly problematic. After a brief exam, his doctor had me take Dad directly to the ER to undergo brain scans. Those revealed a cerebral aneurysm, a weak or thin spot on a blood vessel in Dad's eighty-nine-year-old brain. An aneurysm can put pressure on a nerve or brain tissue and even rupture, spilling blood into the surrounding tissue. This one was growing so rapidly that it now threatened to pressure his brain and push it through the skull. Dad might have had the aneurysm since birth, I was told, but the more likely scenario was that this head trauma occurred during the recent fall. It all sounded unbelievably scary.

Dad's doctor and I quickly consulted several brain surgeons. They advised that unless we allowed him brain surgery, Dad's aneurysm would continue to protrude into the skull and end his life. I was told there were three risks associated with Dad's having brain surgery. The first involved the anesthesia, the second was related to whatever injuries he might suffer from the invasive procedure, and the third involved the challenges of brain surgery and recovery on a man his age. I was told to bring a copy of his do-not-resuscitate (DNR) orders. "Just in case," the doctors said.

I was told that Jack would also need extensive postoperative rehabilitation so he could relearn how to speak, eat, swallow, and otherwise function. Unfortunately, their postsurgical prognosis wasn't much brighter. The doctors weren't certain he could recover successfully, as no one yet knew what his aging brain's limitations to learn "new things" were, how long it might take him to recover functioning, or if he would he ever "come back."

I was filled with questions, and there were few definitive answers. No one really knew. There were simply too many unknown factors. What I did know was that I had no other viable choices, since my father needed the surgery to survive and he needed it now. So, with a heavy heart, I authorized the doctors to shave his head in preparation for brain surgery.

I wanted to concentrate completely on Dad at this time, but I couldn't because, as any parent with more than one child knows, part of us needs to attend to the "other kids," even during an emergency. In my case, Mom also desperately needed me to be there for her. As might be expected, Lillian too was suffering from shock and filled with her own fears and confusion while we were hearing about Dad's condition and proposed treatment.

Mom's reliance on him had been part of their ongoing dynamic—he was the oldest son in his family and she the youngest child—and this reflected how they worked out parts of their relationship. Since Jack's retirement, they'd done just about everything together. And by this point at the ALF, my parents had been spending most of their waking hours in the same room together. They expected to eat together, take walks together, watch the same television programs and be with each other all the time. If Mom needed something opened, Dad was there to open it for her. Even if Dad were hungry for lunch, he'd wait until she was ready to go with him.

During our endless wait for the surgeon to emerge with news of the operation, the woman who'd loved her husband for over sixty years and their only child agonized, sitting in limbo. Anyone who has had to sit in a hospital while a loved one undergoes a complicated and dangerous procedure can appreciate the agony and the fearful imaginings we were experiencing.

I thought of every possible concern. How would Dad's fall impact the rhythm my parents had created in their marriage and now at their facility? What would it be like for Jack to be staying alone in some rehabilitation center after his surgery? Would he be lonely? Disoriented? Would Dad miss his wife and be unable to sleep? Would he ever learn to walk and talk again, or would he spend his remaining days without Mom in continuing decline?

I further worried how Mom would survive her time without him. Would she continue to attend the activities she enjoyed—her chair yoga classes and the bingo games? If Dad remained away long or didn't live beyond the surgery, how badly would Lillian's anxiety interfere with her functioning? Would she make new friends? How much additional attention would Mom need during Dad's rehabilitation? And on and on.

When the surgeon finally emerged hours later, his demeanor was measured and calm. His tone reminded me of Sgt. Friday from the old *Dragnet* TV show: "Just the facts ma'am." I listened to him say he'd successfully removed as much as he safely could and that Dad should make a "decent recovery." I had just begun to breathe more freely when he added: "You know, Jack's brain has been reduced to the size of a walnut from all his dementia." *His* dementia? Oh no! That news really shocked me.

None of Dad's physicians had ever alluded to his having this dreaded affliction. I was trying to process both the cruel image the brain surgeon had drawn for us as well as the long-term consequences of this news when he dealt a second blow. The surgeon actually took a plastic soda bottle out of my mother's hand, pointed to the remains of her drink and said: "I had to take that much fluid out of his head." Unbelievable! Thankfully, I don't think Mom fully understood him. She'd only heard the part that her man would be okay and returning to her, and that made her very happy.

We were permitted a brief visit with him. Lying there attached to monitoring machines, Dad looked smaller and frailer than I'd ever seen him. I could see that his recovery would be arduous. Dad would need rest and then extensive rehabilitation in order to learn to walk and talk again. And I didn't know what, if anything, could be done at this point for Dad's newly reported dementia. I did know that Mom would need me to manage more things for her now that Dad would be unavailable, and I wondered where I'd find the additional time.

According to his surgeon, Dad had a very limited brain, but, according to the hospital's physical therapy staff, it was a teachable brain. Jack remained remarkably cheerful throughout his rehab. He developed this habit of thanking everyone who took care of him, often three times. People at the rehab facility often stopped me in the hall to share their appreciation of Dad's inspiring results and his optimistic attitude. He was willing to allow the doctors to probe and push him without complaint. He took his medicines, food, and water voluntarily and as prescribed. He did his rehab as regularly as he'd done his exercises every morning when I'd been a girl. Dad went through the process with the same resolve I'd seen in him in his younger days. Through rehabilitation, he was able to regain most of his strength and all of his speech.

My Mom did as well as she could without having him by her side to help her stay organized and calm. I saw her more often during the weeks Dad was away recovering. She continued going to meals, of course, and to the activities she liked, and she even started making some new friends. She never complained to me, and only once during Dad's absence was I called in to see the ALF administrator about Lillian's questionable behaviors. Then Jack came back, they were together again, and things went along pretty ordinarily for a little while.

YOUR STORY

Frankly there are limitations on how much permanence you will get or can expect from any of your POPlans, no matter how well thought out they are. Similarly, there are limitations on how much you can protect any other human being, especially another adult, something you've undoubtedly seen. Even with many sets of eyes watching, a frail elderly person can easily take a fall, forget to take the right medication at the right time, or lose a hearing aid in the sheets. Nearly one in three women who are sixty-five years old today will take a fall. One half of those over age eighty-five will fall whether they live at home or in a senior facility.[1]

The consequences of falling can be potentially life changing. Certainly, they'll require you to alter your POPlan. Eighty percent of those in California rehabilitation facilities are there because they took a fall. Of those, 65 percent will never return home. Falls are the most common cause of traumatic brain injuries (TBI).

In 2000 TBI accounted for 46 percent of fatal falls among older adults.[2] People who are seventy-five and older who fall are four to five times more likely than those aged sixty-five to seventy-four to be admitted to a long-term care (LTC) facility for a year or more as a result.[3] Hip fractures are particularly concerning because older people often can't learn to walk again. Thereafter, their prolonged immobility and functional disability put these seniors at even greater risk for additional diseases.

No matter how watchful everyone's eyes and how attentive you are, it seems impossible to prevent all falls and accidents. One of the dangerous and limiting effects for people who've fallen even once is developing the fear of falling. That concern may cause your parents to unduly limit their activities. Ironically, by reducing their mobility, your parents will lose some physical fitness and actually increase their risk of falling.[4] In a moment, on the way back from the bathroom even with a caregiver holding on, your parent can take a fall. No one is immune.

Since I never recommend more oversight of your parents than is necessary, your POP task here, as elsewhere, is determining the right amount of care and oversight. Would more caregiver help have prevented Dad from falling in the bathroom? Probably not, but maybe the caregiver would have walked him to the john? How much oversight might I have needed when Dad's "silent" aneurysm was growing? Hard to say, and maybe no amount of prevention is perfect.

To do more for your aging parents than they need can infantilize and weaken them. If you hire too much caregiving too early or hover over your parents day and night, you may encourage a premature loss of confidence that may lead to many unwanted outcomes, including falling. While some parents do need substantial help, others do not. Anyone can get lazy when there's someone around to do all the lifting. When your aging parents rely on others unnecessarily, their results may include loss of muscle mass, weight gain, diminution of cognitive ability, and of the joy of feeling independent.

How will you know the right amount of attention that your parents need? You won't always know. But to get the best estimate, watch your parents carefully and ask as many of the right questions as possible. Evaluate your parents for something called the "frailty syndrome," a condition primarily due to the age-related loss and dysfunction of muscle and bone. Stay alert to the five most common elements of frailty syndrome: unintentional weight loss, muscle weakness, unexplained exhaustion, low physical activity level, and a slowed walking speed. Those seniors rated most frail on this scale have the greatest potential for harm and need the most attention.

Another thing to do *before* your parents have accidents or take the kinds of falls mine did is to look at whether there are better ways to prevent such events. There are some simple things you can do to lessen the probability of serious falls, like putting down non-stick mats under area rugs, eliminating unnecessary electrical cords and wires and ridding their halls of the attractive nuisance of clutter.

If you've been carefully watching your parents' decline, it's likely you've seen erratic changes. Part of your difficulty in knowing the correct degree of protection your parents need is that it may vary from day to day, even change for the worse after sunset (called "sundowning") or over the course of a single day. Even if they've been diagnosed with some form of dementia or delirium, parts of your parents' brain may still be working fairly well, especially at certain times of day. Your parents also may sometimes dissemble, which can confuse you, or hide things from you. They may be very needy on a Wednesday night but by Friday morning, after a refreshing night's sleep, appear to have changed substantially for the better. Even as you aim to protect them, you'll need to avoid underestimating your parents' abilities.

Each parent has his or her own disabilities and declines at a unique pace. That is part of why your seemingly perfect POPlan may fail. Differing aging patterns alter the dynamics of your parents' lives together, which not only can be stressful in a long marriage with its well-established habits, but may require you to come up with alternative plans you'd never considered.

When one of your parent's geriatric limitations exceeds the other's, everyone involved may feel unsettled. Sometimes one of your parents becomes the caregiver to a more disabled or substantially older spouse. Other times, their divergent conditions require placement in different facilities. You, like me, may have several of these events happen over the course of your POPcycle. You will want to be aware that intense feelings—such as abandonment, survivor guilt, shock, betrayal, and even rage—may arise for the spouse left behind by one who no longer functions well or remembers the other. Ironically it may be a relief as well.

Now that you've come to the point in your POPcycle where you've put in place as many safety measures for your parents' lives, homes, and property, as you can manage and they will tolerate, many of your remaining tasks will simply involve maintenance. You may even have a lot of time on your hands to watch and wait. Ironically, much of your challenge may involve the fact that there's little to fix or do.

Sometimes when you're frustrated because you have nothing POParental to do, you may decide to do something, anything, to "be helpful." You might even find yourself making up things to do for your parents. You may have their swallowing retested to see if they can eat more interesting foods. You may suggest more physical therapy to see if it will lighten your parents' depression or give them more physical challenges through exercise. There may be times when your efforts are relatively fruitless, but you may just want to feel you're doing something useful. To be candid, I did all of those.

When you feel sad that your loved ones are failing in front of your eyes, you may even try to "fix" those things that are already working. You may try to micromanage your parents' care, unconsciously hoping you can regain control over things that feel uncontrollable. Don't change things in your POPlan unless they're not working and you have to. What can you do instead of messing with what's working? You can focus on your gratitude for their health and longevity.

Often there isn't a lot you can do but sit by patiently, be grateful for their aliveness, and enjoy your parents as much as possible in the time you have left with them. There are times when listening to your parents may be the most kind and POParental thing to do. Listen to them respectfully. Pay attention to what your parents say they want or need and to what they don't say. Some days it just plain hurts when the people you looked up to and loved become diminished. But it *is* all part of the Circle of Life. Does that make it hurt any less? Watching and waiting can be oppressive or joy filled. It's up to you.

12

EXPECTING THE UNEXPECTED
WHEN WE'RE DOING POP

MY STORY

Early one morning, a bit later in our POPcycle, I got another significant POP phone call. This time it was from a concerned employee at my parents' assisted-living facility (ALF). Mom had taken a bad fall. She tripped while making the bed I'd erroneously believed was being made for my parents by the staff. Lillian had turned away the first set of medics, refusing their help or to go with them to the hospital. Clearly, a "disciplinarian" POParent was needed on-site. I reassured the staff member that I would come as soon as I could drive there and take care of things. "Please call her another ambulance. I'll be right over and make sure she gets to the hospital."

By the time I arrived, the paramedics had already returned. One was in the bathroom where Mom apparently had "landed" after her fall. Now she was in much pain and "acting out," as therapists say of teenagers. I overheard the brawny professional warning her: "Look lady, I don't care if you are ninety years old, if you don't stop fighting me and let me do my job, I will call the police." He came out to the living room where Dad, the head of the facility, and I all sat demurely. "Is she always this difficult?" he asked. Three heads nodded simultaneously.

As it turned out, my osteoporotic mother had taken a serious fall and damaged her hip. The hip is the body's second-largest bone and is central to all lower-body movement. Within minutes, Lillian was transported to the hospital. The details and sequencing of events in the ER are a blur for me. The combination of stress, super-bright lighting, an endless list of unknowns, and just plain fear generated a feeling of timeless spaciness in my head.

Hence the next thing I recall was coming back to "consciousness" and watching Mom being wheeled away on a gurney, apparently headed for major surgery. I jumped up and started running after them—no one had spoken with me nor gotten my signature on her consent forms. The confused-looking nurse told me: "Lillian said it was fine and told us she had *no* family." Uh-oh.

Mom's postsurgical experience evolved into a far bigger nightmare than earlier that morning. Never a shrinking violet, my mother had seemingly morphed into the patient from hell. In the days following the procedure, Mom's surgeon actually refused to visit her in the hospital, claiming he wouldn't attend a patient who was spitting at and biting him and the hospital staff.

Subsequent to those episodes, my mother mysteriously began refusing both food and water. As a result, she couldn't take her medications and, should it continue, would soon become malnourished. Her decision put the hospital in a legally compromised situation. Since they lacked the legal authority to force her to ingest anything and feared for their liability, the hospital personnel spent hours and hours trying to place Mom in a psychiatric ward, even in a rehabilitation facility—anywhere to get her off their wards.

As that long Saturday afternoon dragged on and no one could locate a single facility in Ventura County willing to accept Lillian Wolf, things began to get desperate. Mom's health was being compromised by her actions and attitudes and it would only get worse with more time.

With the clock ticking away and frustration increasing from all quarters, only one viable option remained. I had to leave the hospital to go get and bring in the Big Guns—Dad. I raced back to the ALF and briefed Dad about our situation in the car as we drove back to the hospital. As he approached his wife, Dad put on his grimmest, most authoritative face and announced that, until she took food, water, and her meds, he would neither talk with nor listen to Mom. That put an immediate end to her boycott. I knew it—Jack still had the power with his wife!

In the long run however, Mom never did really recover from the fall. She never learned to walk on her own again, despite valiant efforts by the long-suffering physical therapists. Even I tried to work with them by holding out my open arms to her, quite literally, during her physical therapy (PT) sessions. Her fear of falling again, the cognitive limitations that made it too hard to learn "new things" or follow directions, her physical weakness, and whatever unknowns all conspired together.

With her life confined to chairs and beds, not surprisingly, my formerly weight-conscious Mom gained pounds easily, became less mentally alert, and grew more depressed. Unable to follow through with the demands of PT, Medicare soon cut off that option, and Mom's once graceful body became forever limp. Several people would be needed thereafter to lift and transfer her.

Clearly Mom's returning to the ALF would not be possible. From a financial point of view, we couldn't afford the monthly expense of two full-time caregivers on top of paying for ALF for both of them. Nor was the ALF viable from the point of view of the level of care she was beginning to require, which was readily provided in a skilled nursing facility (SNF).

Jack's physical, cognitive, and emotional needs didn't require the same level of care that Mom's did. He chose to stay at the AL, where he was comfortable, and he began to create a life there by himself. Although his world had become smaller in a way, Dad seemed to thrive, reading his books—sometimes over and again—watching his TV shows, and sharing himself with only a few. I saw that he craved the peace and quiet he'd not had living with Mom, for a long time—perhaps since their beginning together.

Frankly, he seemed somewhat relieved. Dad enjoyed the role of being called in to rescue Mom, comfort her, and visit with her. Without having to share space with anyone, Jack took the opportunity to create his "man cave" of books, television, and occasionally some music.

My Mom's life would thereafter be spent alone, too, but differently than Dad's. After her fall, like so many older people, Mom lacked what she needed to regain most of her previous life. My parents' married life together, as they'd known it for over sixty years was over, and I witnessed her life becoming even more limited and frail. It was very sad.

YOUR STORY

One of the most challenging jobs as a POParent is to get proficient at managing the unexpected, whatever its source. What caused my family's POPlans to be dismantled won't be the same things that disrupt your POPlans. Your family will need to use its available resources to address your parents' unplanned-for happenings and the further consequences of those events, and then to craft its own unique, workable solutions. Nonetheless a common theme emerges for all POParents: how can you plan for the unexpected when you're doing POP?

The term "snafu" is attributed to the American military from the Second World War. The initial letters stand for "systems normal, all fouled up." If you're doing POP, snafus are probably an everyday occurrence. Your ability to remain flexible and resilient, to not crumble when things don't go as expected is—and will remain—one of your most important qualifications for doing this job satisfyingly. Like all POParents you'll do a better job when you're willing—and able—to face what's ahead with candor and objectivity rather than fantasy and wishful thinking.

Even if you can't predict exactly when or why snafu's will occur, you can: predict they will; have some fall-back POPlans, and work on how to regain your equilibrium as quickly as possible after they descend. You also can get better at managing your emotions and yourself when these unexpected events do occur. Finally, you can learn to get better at resetting your family's POPcycle back on a useful course as quickly as possible when your POPlans get interrupted.

Tragically your aging parents may have been let down by one (or more) of the many institutions originally set up to protect them—Medicare, Social Security, insurers, their ALF, and so on. In some cases you may find yourself facing three "Goliaths." Each of these behemoths may be staffed with lots of experienced people who have time to get things done, whereas you, "David" here, may be extremely limited in terms of your experience, time, and energy.

You may also be frustrated by fussy parents who may be confused by these various entities, want something special, or don't want to go where you've found them the "perfect" place. It's insulting and disappointing that the profit motive has so often trumped private institutional caring and how often governmental agencies have disappointed the elderly and disabled. You may find yourself seeking solutions to complex situations where it feels like you're navigating a course between the proverbial rock and a hard place—one institution, say Medicare, on one side and another institution, your parents' physician perhaps, on the other.

You and your siblings may be scratching your heads, figuring out how to keep your own paying jobs, health, and marriages while also performing your POP miracles. Hopefully, you won't need to get your dad a timely admission to an appropriate placement (one corporation and its rules) before the hospital (a second giant institution) sends him home, having been pressured financially by Medicare (a third institution) to release the patient quickly. In any case, you will likely encounter your own challenges with "rocks" and "hard places."

POParents can't expect these often overburdened institutions to always be advocates for your parents. You'll have to discover what you need to know about these organizations and how they work (or don't work). Doing so will be imperative for helping your aging loved ones through this part of their life. You will need to recognize that this arena is one of shifting sands legislatively and administratively.

As a result, you can rarely learn all you need to know in advance of needing to know it. You must jump in and immerse yourself whenever a POP problem needs solving, which is considerably easier now than it was in years past because of the internet, social networking, and POP's home website, as we'll talk more about in this book's final chapter.

It is useful for POParents to be conversant with the most common ways the seniors in your charge may become weakened or even die unexpectedly. You'll want to be conversant with the diseases your parents may be particularly vulnerable to, but you need not become familiar with every geriatric disorder nor obsess that your parents will come down with one or more of them just because they're advanced in age.

To pay proper POP attention to a disease or disorder, you'll need to be aware of its most common symptoms. So, for example, if your parents have had pneumonias and you hear them coughing persistently for days, you'll want to take them to the doctor. Pneumonia is one of the leading causes of death among seniors and the leading cause of morbidity and mortality among those seniors who live in long-term care (LTC) facilities.

Over the course of our POPcycle, my parents came down with pneumonia so frequently that I lost count. During their California years, pneumonia was the cause of every hospitalization for both my parents, except for the consequences of their taking falls. I had hoped to be able to better protect Mom and Dad from the ravages of pneumonia in balmy Southern California, but that didn't prove to be the case. Pneumonia also is the primary reason that residential facilities, like ALFs and board and cares (B&Cs) transfer their residents to more acute locations, like SNFs and hospitals. Other symptoms of pneumonia include fever; fatigue; loss of appetite; discomfort in the chest, lungs, or upper abdomen; discolored sputum (green or bloody phlegm); and disorientation. Take your parents to competent professionals for diagnosis and treatment, especially if their coughs or runny nose appear to be chronic.

Physicians often rely on reported clinical changes (physical, functional, or mental) in an older patient's status to signal that something may be wrong, since pneumonia can be difficult to diagnose and X-rays are not always helpful. But because your elderly parents often lack good memories, they aren't always useful as their own medical historians. They may lose track of how long they've had their symptoms. Your aging parents may also wish to avoid yet another trip to the doctor for "just a cough." When asked about their cough or runny nose, your parents might say: "I don't like to complain, honey." Therefore it will become even more your POP responsibility to pay attention to symptoms that persist.

There are two distinct types of pneumonia: community-acquired and aspiration pneumonia. Community-acquired pneumonia is airborne and easily communicable, thus presenting major challenges both during cold winters and in senior facilities, where the large number of people present may support quick contagion. Seniors often arrive at facilities with their immune systems and swallowing functions already compromised due to age and preexisting medical conditions (such as a stroke, congestive heart failure, or other disorders).

There are some steps you can take to prevent the spread of community-acquired pneumonia, influenza, and colds. You can remind your parents to wash their hands frequently with sanitizers or other substances that stop the spread of bacteria. You can easily and economically sanitize handles on their shopping carts at the market and on their light switches, door handles, and window handles at home. You can ascertain if your parents' phones and any community computers they touch are sanitized. Similarly, if your parents use keyboards in public places like the library, you can recommend ways to clean them thoroughly beforehand. You and your parents can avoid using public telephones, especially in emergency rooms. You might also urge your parents to forgo reading magazines in doctors' offices, where many sick people may have fingered them. Instead, bring along your own periodicals, tablet, iPad, and the like to amuse your folks, show them your photos, and play games with them while you wait.

The second type is aspiration pneumonia. It develops from a combination of factors that may include fairly common things such as impaired swallowing, fluids draining into their lungs, and inhaling bacteria from the back of their throat, mouth, or nose into the lungs. Preventing your parents from getting aspiration pneumonia is possible, but it will require your parents to change some of their habitual ways. That is not easy and it's far from foolproof. You can begin by altering your parents' diet so it consists primarily of softer foods that are easier to swallow. You can also give them a thickener to add into their liquids and perhaps you (or an occupational therapist) can teach your parents new swallowing maneuvers.

The treatment for pneumonia is generally straightforward, typically lasts ten to fourteen days, and doesn't depend on how the disease was contracted. Initially, antibiotics are administered to kill the bacteria. With this illness, as with others, you will want to check that your parents are receiving the correct geriatric dosages of medications. A senior's body often requires or can handle only smaller amounts of prescription drugs. Breathing treatments and expectorants are also frequently introduced to open up their airways, loosen phlegm, and cough out the mucus that accompanies pneumonia. Some of the most serious hazards are caused when your parents lie flat in bed all day, because fluids tend to settle into their lungs.

Seniors with pneumonia in just one part of their lungs have a good chance of full recovery. The presence of pneumonia in several parts of the lungs is more severe and makes recovery more difficult. With advancing age, the lung tissue becomes less elastic, decreasing the lung's ability to expand and contract. Even osteoporosis, another common geriatric disorder, with its resulting deformity and curvature of the spine can affect breathing by impairing lung expansion.

Your POP responsibility includes helping your parents avoid all predictable health risks, just as your parents did for you when you were young. You'll need to research and weigh the advantages and disadvantages of having your parents receive pneumococcal and influenza vaccines. Many geriatric professionals believe that because seniors' bodies are more vulnerable than other adults, everyone over sixty-five should be inoculated against such diseases. Others hold differing views. If you've hired professionals you trust and they think a course of treatment is best for your parents, you'll want to follow much of their advice. If you find you are consistently not aligned with your parents' physicians' point of view or you aren't taking their advice, find other doctors with whom you can work in better accord.

One health hazard for your senior parents that may surprise you is being admitted as a patient to a hospital. Hospitals concentrate lots of people with serious health problems into small spaces. Many POParents attempt to keep their parents out of the hospital unless it's absolutely necessary. When I'd visit one sick parent in the hospital, I'd keep the other parent at home, rather than expose my healthy parent to a lot of sick patients.

Some of their hospitalizations caused my parents unforeseen complications. I was told that my Mom had contracted a case of Methicillin-resistant Staphylococcus aureus (MRSA) during one such hospitalization. MRSA is a bacterium that can be fatal. Sometimes it is called the "superbug" because it is resistant to many commonly used antibiotics. It weakens the immune system of those already vulnerable physically and it's rampant in some hospitals. When I would visit Mom in the hospital after she got MRSA, I had to wear a mask, a gown, and other protective clothing. Later on, when I would need to place my mother again in other SNFs, some refused to admit her because she carried the contagious disorder.

Generally speaking, parents who reside in LTC facilities have higher levels of functional disability and underlying medical illness than their peers who live out in the community. I was unaware of that fact when I placed my parents in such residences. I also didn't consider that some contagious diseases would spread more easily in these facilities. However, as I like to tell my patients, we must make all decisions with "inadequate information," and nonetheless, we must decide. Looking back, I still wouldn't have changed my POP choices, since they seemed wise when I made them, and I felt that I had done the best I could when I made those choices.

Some estimate that, in the near future, as many as 40 percent of Americans will spend some time living in a LTC facility. Given our baby boomer demographics, it's foreseeable that the number of frail older adults living in these facilities (including ALFs, SNFs, and B&Cs) will increase dramatically over the next thirty years. Some POP families may find community-based options preferable to LTC facilities. But as responsible POParents, it's important that you not overreact to every potential danger or jump to hasty and unwarranted generalizations. Whether or not the results turn out as you expected, as good POParents, you must decide things sanely and thoughtfully, considering all the elements available to you at the time.

13

TURNING POP INTO
OUR GIANT DO-OVER

Forgiveness, Compassion, and
Gratitude Fill the Space

MY STORY

I fondly recall "do-overs" from my childhood. In those days, my aunts, uncles, cousins, and a myriad of kids would regularly congregate at the midtown "penthouse playground" where my favorite cousin Rick and his parents lived. It was a New York City child's Disneyland. Spanning over the whole building, their penthouse home had endless rooms and space outdoors for us to play in. Their roof patio was so vast that we could even lose our parents there, and I think they got the chance to lose us kids, too.

A Ping-Pong table dominated the entryway, and it was always a major attraction for me. Often the adults and children would play round-robin table tennis, where each team would race around the table trying to score points. In my family and maybe in yours, if one of the children shouted "do-over!" while playing a game, she or he would be allowed to take a second turn.

A rule that permitted do-overs seemed ironic, offering my young mind food for thought. I remember contemplating that the world would be a less harsh and more magnanimous place if we could all try again when our first attempts weren't all we'd hoped they would be. The rule was grounded in an underlying optimism—if we were given another chance, we'd play better the second time than we did the first. The do-over rule seemed a beacon of hope, suggesting a universe where there was fairness and flexibility for those less able—in that case, small children.

I began to wonder: Could there be "do-overs" in life? And, why should only young people get them? Why couldn't everyone be afforded such a compassionate opportunity to perform better or get a more desirable result? As I continued to ponder these ideas, I also warmed to the rule when I saw that it actually allowed for and encouraged forgiveness. If my first time didn't have to count and I were able to try again, I might be forgiven my bumbling first attempts at certain things. Surely that kind of forgiveness would moderate some of life's harsher moments.

What if everyone could revisit parts of their life and call for a do-over to produce more desirable outcomes? What if we were given the option for do-overs in our relationships with our spouses, parents, children, and siblings? Wouldn't we all want to obtain a few do-overs now and again? Or would such a more forgiving rule discourage people from doing their best the first time out? Couldn't it supply a handy excuse for people's bad behaviors?

I mulled over these questions and then asked myself an important philosophical question. What if we could all have a greater chance for happiness the second time around with some life do-overs? Wouldn't that be more humane?

Years later, when I became a psychotherapist, I again considered the possible implications for healing: would we be healthier and perhaps more peaceful were we able to invoke a do-over consciousness but also do that responsibly and thoughtfully. What if we were given something like a second chance to do over parts of the past and, this time, we could possess the understanding, knowledge, sensibilities, and skills we have now? Who among us wouldn't want the chance to be a better parent to our kids? Or a better friend to someone we may have let down? Maybe even those people who've treated us unkindly would want a do-over too?

Periodically I ask my patients a question that, at this point in the POPcycle, I asked myself as well: if you could wave a magic wand and improve something from your past, what do-over might you choose? My purpose in accessing regrets, as the question does, is to inform ourselves about our current values. What are things we hold dear today that we may not have demonstrated as much in the past? What might we have done better, with a do-over?

One answer that came to mind was: Could I be a more loving daughter or a more devoted POParent if given a second chance? What if there were a way to "reverse time" so I could try parenting again, now as a more mature and compassionate person? What if POP could give me that chance?

As I matured, I had often found myself admiring and even emulating many of my parents' qualities. And as I began taking on the challenges of raising young stepchildren, I often tried to borrow these parental qualities. Now I had even gotten the chance to become the "mother" that Lillian had said I was.

One of the qualities I emulated was my parents' determination to get results. Even those first days of POP, I'd insisted upon taking Mom to not one but two doctors and thereafter to the hospital to get answers and treatment for them. My mother and father had done the same for me when I was the child.

Dogged pursuit was a parental quality I had learned, perhaps copied, from my parents. I remembered their tireless quests for whatever I needed. They vigorously searched for those things, whether it was a book for a class assignment, a doctor with the answers to some mysterious condition, or the right matching blouse for my camp uniform. Sometimes, to avoid their intensity, I wouldn't even ask my parents for something. Maybe this makes sense solely to an only child, but two tall parents with their intense

pursuit can be overwhelming to a youngster, and that hadn't always been easy for me.

When raising me, they'd encouraged my young brain to keep
learning and expanding: another of their parental qualities that I
had valued and sought to emulate as my way to "pay them back."
With my do-over and me as the POP Mom, I aimed to discover
how to similarly promote continued development in their aging
brains and bodies.

They'd also been very generous parents, Lillian and Jack, sharing all they had: their time, their love, and themselves with me.
Now with this do-over, I asked myself if I could show my parents
even more generosity and benevolence in my POParent role than
I'd yet shown them or even my kids? The second time around,
now as the POParent, could I do even better?

If I could parent Lillian and Jack with the best of what I was
today (the more mature, spiritual woman I'd tried to become)
maybe they would receive better POParenting from me now than
the parenting my step-kids had gotten decades before. Now I
possessed more patience, compassion, and even more humor than
years before. Maybe at this point in my journey, I could do an
even better job POParenting Lillian and Jack than they'd done
parenting me. What a crazy thought that was!

I felt that POP clearly held the potential to be transformative
for all involved, from the senior generation to the POParents and
to the growing generations of grandchildren and beyond, as well.
As I more immediately anticipated my parents' mortal end and my
own, I saw even more clearly than ever: participating in a POPcyle
was as likely to expand and enlighten us as becoming a parent was!

To act as lovingly and generously as I wanted meant discovering the place in my heart where I was whole and unconditionally
accepting of these two people I'd chosen to POParent. My years of
counseling and spiritual work had shown me that to know that
kind of love, I'd need to place forgiveness at the entryway to my
heart.

To become a nonjudgmental and consistently generous POParent, I would need to repair whatever wounds still remained un-

healed from my own childhood. I began to envision how to do that, create a clean slate. I wished to discover if—and how—I could use all my thoughts and feelings, even the unwanted ones like sadness, anger, and abandonment, in support of these goals. I understood that the road to the kind of loving state I hoped to offer them and myself was through forgiveness.

As odd as it sounds, I saw that I would need to forgive my parents—for just being human and making those mistakes that parents often make. At some time, all parents neglect, scold, embarrass, or even reject their offspring. My parents had, and when I was parenting, I too did some of those things. To be able to lovingly and fully POParent them now, I saw I'd need to forgive my parents for doing whatever "unfortunate things" they'd done all those years ago.

It wasn't long before I saw that there was someone else I'd need to forgive first. I would need to forgive myself even before I sought to forgive my Mom and Dad. I had learned over time that, when we do work on forgiveness, the first party needing forgiveness is, interestingly enough, ourselves. Forgiveness has been called "an inside job" because, after taking inventory of all our acts of commission and omission, it's ourselves we must forgive first before we can truly forgive anyone else. Why? I have my theories but can't say for sure. What I can say is that witnessing this happen hundreds of times has warranted the conclusion: forgiveness starts with ourselves.

I knew that to become the POParent I aspired to be I'd need to discover how to forgive myself—and thereafter my folks. How would I go about this process of forgiving myself? Taking an inventory, as people do in their Twelve-Step recovery programs,[1] was a helpful beginning. I focused on revisiting the ways I'd disappointed myself, the times I'd lost my way. It wasn't a comfortable activity, looking my personal history straight in the eye, the parts I liked and those I didn't. Nonetheless, I aimed to stay with it. I also asked myself if there were parts I could mend? I considered: were there people I could apologize to? Things I could now fix? When the answer was yes, most of the time I would go off and do those things.

At other times it was more difficult to forgive myself. Maybe I'd see a pattern that was self-destructive or that hurt others and I'd want to judge myself for it or defend myself by denying it or attributing the responsibility to someone else. After more work, I had a refreshing and energizing revelation: all my acts of commission and all my omissions, the good and the bad, all I'd ever experienced had led me to today. I'd become who I was today as a result of all my experiences and how I'd interpreted them. Rather than cursing the parts I regretted or resented, I could try to be thankful for how they'd served me. I really could forgive myself.

When I finally got that, I was able to magnanimously forgive myself. Thereafter, I was able to forgive Lillian and Jack of any residual blame I'd held onto from past hurts. I was able to "absolve" my parents for things they'd done or not done in my upbringing. When I could do that, it became unnecessary to hold on to any historic faultfinding. After going through all of that, forgiving anyone else became much easier.

To be a good POParent, it was love I wanted to feel and hold onto, not old resentments. I wanted to feel and act compassionately toward those who'd given me life. Holding on to those past hurts really made little sense. It got in the way of my being the loving person and POParent I wanted to be. In any case, Lillian and Jack could hardly remember breakfast, let alone any harm they may have caused me fifty years ago. Retaining unresolved thoughts and feelings from the past only interfered with my ability to love my folks—and myself—in the present.

Invoking my compassion through my intention to be lovingly POParental and my process of forgiveness, I came to notice that I was filled with gratitude. I would experience being grateful for having my two parents alive. I was grateful I could provide them loving attention. When I could sit long enough to bask in the gratitude, my mind would often reward me with positive recollections. Triggering happy memories gave me the chance to consciously savor the good times I had shared with my family and reminded me there could be more of those in the future.

Happiness scientists report that focusing our attention on three activities will provide the most useful basis for expanding our happiness. These activities are forgiveness, gratitude, and savoring the good in life. Being able to do each of these while facing the challenges of POParenting can be hard work, but I was observing that such efforts could bring much joy to me and my family.

Because I was also doing my work with these activities, it became easier to recognize that POP was not only "a good thing" for a family member to do for a senior, but also POP was a remarkable opportunity for transformation and healing as well as responsibility and worry. When I saw I could use the whole POPcycle as my own giant do-over, I realized how much participating in it could boost my personal growth. The unexpected result of parenting my own parents could turn out to be my own personal expansion. And once I saw that so clearly, I knew I would eventually need to share these lessons and this realization with others. Then others who were still feeling as alone and burdened as I once had felt doing POP could also feel the freedom, love, and joy—the extraordinary transformative potential of POParenting.

Thereafter, I noticed that I'd begun to act more patiently with my folks, more compassionately than I ever had previously. My heart was opened to feeling things in new ways. I was finally able to put myself in the shoes of my parents, to understand Their Story more fully. I felt more deeply what each of them was going through as they headed toward their final days on the planet. Maybe I just could become the unconditionally loving parent to Lillian and Jack that I'd always wanted them to be to me?

In spite of all this work I did on myself, some days the emotional and practical demands of doing POP alone, without any siblings to support me or help make decisions, seemed too vast to manage. If it took a village to raise a child, I thought, how many does it take to raise a parent? Especially during this part of the POPcycle when I felt so unable to control aspects of my parents' lives, I revived an old childhood daydream about having a sibling.

As an only child I'd often found myself wanting a sibling, some-one to help me with perspective on our parents. None arrived. My most recurring fantasy was of having an older brother, someone to protect me—although I wasn't entirely sure from what—and someone to hang out with me, although, in truth, older brothers rarely want to do that. I used to imagine that with a brother I would have someone "on my side" in the child-parent dynamic, and life would feel less lonely, even when I also saw how siblings could mistreat one another and act out of jealousy or competition instead of protecting one another.

At this time in our POPcycle, I found myself having similar daydreams about a sibling to make my POP life easier: we'd co-POParent. I would have more help. I could share the burdens of decision-making. I'd have a brother or sister to hang out with me while we did POP together, and protect me—from what, I again didn't know.

Then my logical left-brain returned to poke some holes in my fantasy of co-POParenting. No one could protect me from the hardest part—my parents' inevitable deaths that lay ahead. No sibling, friend, or lover could do my healing work for me. Whether or not I had siblings, it was only I who could practice forgiveness, bring more gratitude for all I'd been given, and savor the wonders of my life. Only I could do these things for myself.

I further considered that there could be a downside to having sisters or brothers when POParenting. I'd need to consult with them on POP, or they with me. We'd need to reach a consensus on every important POP decision. What if we didn't? That could present its own challenges.

In my program of POP Family Coaching, I teach that co-POParenting with some siblings is far from stress free. I've seen firsthand how having siblings co-POParent can sometimes be far harder than doing it solo. By their nature, siblings always contrib-ute divergent amounts of time, money, attention, skills, and other resources. The most positive way to see that is that everyone brings different things to POParenting, enriching the collective effort with their unique contributions. But different ways of contributing can be a source of family feuds, especially when some family members ascribe a negative meaning to those inequities.

The most common form of feuding occurs after POParenting is over and siblings fight over their parents' possessions. I've witnessed feelings that had been dormant and unresolved possibly for decades get stirred up in this process. As a result, hurtful protracted litigation and further family divisions have sometimes ensued.

When I weighed some of the advantages of being a sole POParent versus one with siblings, I realized that, despite looking good from the outside, co-POParenting carries its own burdens. There is no ideal formula for POP satisfaction.

Nonetheless, I still felt an emotional longing to have a sibling. I decided that I didn't want to live the remainder of my POPcycle or my own senior years without someone in the role of my sibling. I told those I counseled that if you want something enough in this lifetime, go out and get it—so long as you don't hurt others along the way. Why couldn't that apply to me about having a sibling? What did it matter that my parents were ninety years old and had long lost their reproductive capabilities? Why couldn't I adopt a brother or a sister because I wanted one?

Presumably, any sibling I'd want would already have a strong affiliation with me, probably would have shared my childhood memories and known me back in the day. I hoped that someone would also share my spiritual point of view, live in the same state, and be intrigued to have a new sibling of their own.

Immediately I thought of Rick, my favorite cousin, whose amazing "penthouse playground" had been my second home when we were growing up. Of all the cousins I'd been close with, he and I, two only children, had always been closest to each other. We'd always stayed involved in each other's lives as we grew into adults, parents, and then POParents. Rick had moved his family from Texas to California in order to POParent my Aunt Molla, when she'd needed his loving attention a while back.

I sat down and wrote to Rick, proposing that we adopt each other as brother and sister and then awaited his reply to my unique request with some apprehension. Rick, of course, thought it a great idea, but we did kind of think alike!

Once onboard, Rick and I collaborated on what language our sibling agreement would contain and how we'd "formalize" it. We decided to perform a little reciprocal adoption ritual we designed, where we made pledges of sibling love and caring and invited a friend to bear witness. The ceremony was officiated by Rick and me on his patio at sunset where we'd said our few lovely words of commitment to each other. Afterward, we three drank a glass of bubbly in celebration.

Although we did nothing to give it any official recognition, our sibling relationship has been recognized in our hearts since that day. The adoption was never about expecting the other to take on any financial or other responsibilities for each other. Rather, it was a sweet statement about our being family. It added a new level of affection between Rick and me.

As I observed my parents becoming less and less present at this point in their POPcycle, adopting Rick gave me a sense of being less alone on the planet. Having this new brother added to my feeling rooted at the very time when my original family roots would soon be pulled up from the earth. The ceremony had also been my way of becoming a more loving parent to the Jane whose parents weren't going to be able to protect her or themselves much longer.

I'd spent much of my time and energy at work supporting others and helping them to get what they wanted—whether it was to do something or to have something. I loved that my work afforded me so many opportunities to do that, and I considered it a real privilege. Acquiring a long-sought older brother in my fifties did seem like an unusual accomplishment. Effectuating this adoption gave me the chance to feel good about supporting myself and added to my optimism that we all can create solutions for what we decide we want and need, however unconventional those solutions might be.

It was during this part of our POPcycle when Lillian was having a particularly lucid day that I decided to tell her I'd started writing this book. It is an odd thing about people who suffer from dementia, as any POParent with a demented loved one knows; occasionally, they act like their old selves, but, within a few hours or sometimes even within the same conversation, they disappear into some netherworld all their own. Even though we understood that phenomenon, the speed of those transitions and inconsistencies in behavior and comprehension were confusing to those of us who loved Lillian, and sometimes it was downright painful.

I felt apprehensive telling Mom about this book. I wondered if she'd be able to understand the concept of POP. Would she be able to relate to the irony of our roles having changed or grasp the potential for how others could be helped through a book about POP? However silly or retro it may seem to want our parents to feel proud of us, we probably never get over it. I really wanted my mother to know about the book and what I'd been doing. And, after all, it was Lillian who had been the first to see it and name it POP, in a way—calling me her mother at the ER that night, oh so long ago.

A part of me wondered if Lillian might berate me, when she heard I was writing a book about our life: I imagined she might say: "You're parenting *me*? How dare you say such a thing? I knew you before you were in diapers." But that wasn't at all how she reacted.

I was both relieved and inspired by her response: "Why, honey, that's so wonderful! You're writing a book about parenting parents. I always said I loved how you wrote. And you know, Jane, parents are always working in their children's best interest. Now that I can see you're parenting Jack and me—and helping others to better parent their parents—I feel reassured. I know you'll always do your best for Daddy and me. And reaching out to help other families, that's my girl!"

The day I told Mom about POP and this book, she asked me lots of questions. After a while, she looked up and very genuinely, even innocently, asked: "Where did you *ever* come up with the wonderful idea that you're parenting your parents?" I gulped, not really knowing what to say and through newly forming tears, I told

her: "I got the idea from you, Mom, and I thank you for it." But by
then she again had drifted away.

YOUR STORY

No one gets out of childhood unscathed. At one time or another
anyone who's parented a youngster has been too busy or tired to
listen, has reacted too quickly or overreacted to events. No parent
raises each child exactly right every day of the year. Put another
way, all parents including POParents make mistakes.

And all children feel let down in some way or at some time by
their parents, no matter how well treated they are. Each of you,
like I, had times during your youth when you felt disappointed,
abandoned, neglected, or rejected by your parents, even if their
view of those incidents differs dramatically from your own. And
since feelings are subjective and personal to each one, you can feel
abandoned, neglected, and rejected even when the facts don't
necessarily say you were.

As you've looked back over your growing up, it's likely you have
created a narrative, whether or not you're aware of it. The narrative is a shorthand way to explain to yourself and others "what's
happened to me," from your point of view. To compose it, you
picked out some key examples that illustrated and then confirmed
your viewpoint from among the hundreds of possible memories
you have of your childhood.

One way to see your own narrative is that it might be the story
you traditionally tell someone new, maybe on your second or third
date, about your past dating history. It might be something you
share with a seatmate on a long plane ride. Most people, perhaps
you too, further solidify the "truth" of their narratives by retelling
it, until, after a while, you believe your version *is* the truth, forgetting that others who lived through the same situations construe
them differently.

If your personal narrative includes the fact that your childhood
was damaged because of self-centered parents who didn't care

about your needs, the memories you'll find will bear witness to that. You'll easily recall incidents when your Mom and Dad disregarded you while lavishing gifts and attention on themselves. By contrast, if you viewed your parents as self-sacrificing people, your narrative is likely to be filled with incidents that corroborate those parental qualities.

It's not pathological and, in fact, it's quite natural to consider and remember your experiences from your own perspective. However, you'll want to remember that, since your narrative is self-constructed, you can always write a different, more positive version of your narrative. You wrote it in the first place, so you can write a better one. It turns out that the way you organize your narrative proves to be quite important because it reflects how you see yourself and, in turn, how you're likely to interpret events that occur during your life.

Some of you were given a bushel full of lemons during childhood. If your early years were harsh, hopefully you've taken away many life lessons and been able to "make lots of lemonade." You might have seen that time as victimizing you, leaving you damaged. Or you might interpret those years as strength-building, explaining why and how you became the competent and powerful adult you are today. Those who suffered because of difficult parents or childhoods also had the benefits of learning much-needed survival and resiliency skills early on rather than later in life.

Sometimes your version of you may not reflect how others see you or may be outdated. For example, your narrative may still portray you as a victim of numerous abusive relationships since childhood. But since then, you may have worked on yourself and now see those experiences as lessons and training tools. Because you and others perceive you now very differently from that old story, your narrative needs to be updated. Your self-esteem and the perceptions of others have changed your viewpoint, so your new narrative should focus on you as a strong and resilient person who's learned to survive, even thrive, despite difficult odds, not the vulnerable child you once were.

Your narrative has the potential to either expand or limit you. It can restrict you if you automatically reach the same life conclusions, no matter the circumstances, and don't allow yourself to see yourself and the present as different from the past. Your narrative can also expand you when you use it to guide you to more positively interpret what's happened to you or more accurately attribute meaning to your experiences.

As a way to look at recomposing your old narrative, I'd like to encourage you, as I do my patients, to examine what you'd like said about you at your funeral, what epitaph you might like on your tombstone. When you try on that view of your life, you often see that your older narrative no longer suits who you've become and how you'd like to live out the remainder of your days.

It may be that the very act of composing a new narrative will support your having a more positive view and therefore making wiser choices. For example, rather than belaboring the pain, drama, and blame of years ago when people "done you wrong," your new narrative can reflect your forgiveness and strengths in the face of adversity.

You can choose to forgive your parents and let the past just be complete and over. How can you do that? Each of you will find your own way to achieve that highly desirable goal. You may seek counsel from your faith, a spiritual guide you trust, or from the many books that concentrate on achieving forgiveness. You may do your work by attending workshops, going on retreats alone or with your POP family, or sitting at home with your computers and phones unplugged. Whatever it takes, find your particular route to more emotional freedom. It will be worth the effort. I've shared my techniques and offer you additional tools intended to help you become more forgiving and loving in your POP role (and wherever else you'd like to apply it).

If you choose the path of forgiveness, you'll be heading away from many destructive and, frankly, self-destructive feelings. By releasing undesired grudges, hurts, memories, and misunderstandings from the past, you'll head toward more productive and satisfying times ahead. But be aware that everyone in your environment may not be as forgiving as you, and when you opt to release old negativity about yourself and others, you may be fighting an uphill battle in the highly litigious society twenty-first-century America you live in.

If you buy the original premise of this section that all parenting is flawed, maybe those of you who've had difficulty up until now can also forgive and let go of the pain you believe your parents inflicted on you. If you can, let go of your residual blame, fault-finding, and judging of your family and yourself. If you do, it's likely you'll be able to experience POP with a new lightness of being. Perhaps you'll have emptied out enough emotional toxicity to create the space for a new kind of reconciliation and authentic happiness in your POP family.

Releasing your past hurts means living with more peacefulness, cooperation, and joy in the present. That is a truth many can embrace, even if only as a wise thought. The aim here, after you've released your past wounds about your folks, is to have that peace become your experience during POP. Practicing forgiveness can remove your sense of obligation and help your joy and compassion emerge more fully.

The POParents I've coached consistently report empowering reactions to doing this type of emotional housecleaning. They have far more energy. They say they feel less worn down and more available to do POP in the present moment, as it's occurring. Maybe even more significantly, they experience a kind of softening, feeling a new capability to do POP in a more positive and life-affirming way. With what you're learning here, you too will hopefully be freed up to focus loving attention on your parents rather than on your unresolved issues.

If you have siblings, consider how your POP family can avoid the predictable pitfalls that have divided others. During the stresses of a POPcycle, unresolved issues from childhood may often reappear, even ones you'd thought were resolved long ago. If they do resurface, one or more siblings may aggravate the old wound. A common way you may see that is someone assigns a false meaning to something in the present although what's really going on is that

something still hurts from the past. Your unresolved family dynamics may sound like a lot of things and perhaps like this: "No
wonder you don't want Mom living in the nursing home I chose
for her, right down the street from me. You were her favorite child
and were always jealous when Mom paid any attention to me. Now
you think I'll get to see her more and that's why you don't like the
home I chose."

Sibling rivalry takes many forms and, unfortunately, has no age
limit. In one family a POP daughter may carry residual resentment
that her brother always got the "fun" jobs at home during childhood while she had to do more domestic chores. Now co-
POParenting with her brother, she may insist on keeping all the
"fun" POP tasks, leaving her brother to change diapers and empty
bedpans. In another POP family, two sons might compete for who
will take their mother to the doctor's office, each bearing the
unconscious notion of one-upping the other with superior information.

Speaking of old programming, some of your family may have
the belief that caring for old parents is "women's work." That is
belied by current statistics. In many families, and perhaps yours,
POParenting is regularly being done by sons and sons-in-law as
well as daughters and daughters-in-law.[2] In some families, the
POP work done by siblings is not based along gender lines, whereas in others, there may be a division of roles based on sex. In the
latter, sons and sons-in-law may primarily be involved in POP
banking, financial management, and legal matters while females
are making meals, washing dishes, and changing diapers. In other
POP families where there may be no daughters to do the more
personal tasks, there may be daughters-in-law who attend to those,
paid help, or even the sons may take on such intimate tasks.

POP work divisions among siblings may find their roots either
in your culture's expectations of men and women or in early family
roles seen in your home. If you and your siblings aim to equalize
POP tasks and democratize POP decision-making, it's likely you'll
find it easier to deal with each other, unless your traditions strongly dictate otherwise. That type of equalization and demonstration

of respect can heal siblings' lifelong resentments and inequities, as well as serve your aging parents more appropriately in today's world.

After you've become aware of your issues and done your forgiveness work, a part of healing involves the fun part of visioning—creating the new life or changes you want to have. By way of example, you too can choose a sibling at any age. Any of you who were raised as only children and still yearn for one as I did, or if your siblings have died and you don't wish to go through your POP days, your older days or any more days without a brother or sister, you can do something about that. Although my qualifications for a sibling included someone who remembered me from childhood, that need not be one of your criteria. Anyone can be an eligible candidate so long as each of you desires to make the other a part of your family.

The sibling adoption between Rick and me was not a legal adoption, in the sense that we filed no papers and ultimately there were no legal consequences. Others who choose this "feeling" step may wish to draw up legal wills to leave the "sibling" a portion of his or her property at death. You may find it comforting to exchange other legal documents or responsibilities with your new sibling, such as giving that person your durable health care proxy or your power of attorney. This may be especially helpful if you're single and feeling scared of being "alone" when your parents die.

When I heard Mom tell me that I was "doing good" as her POParent and that she could now "rest comfortably," I loved it. It didn't matter that she had cognitive issues or that I was way over twenty-one, it just felt good. Some of your parents may not express their approval or gratitude all that often—and some maybe continue to grumble—but you should know that they really are grateful. You may need to remind yourself periodically that in spite of your uncertainties and challenges, your aging parents are truly relieved that you noticed they needed help and stepped up to make their lives better by doing POP.

You may feel that you're motivated to POParent primarily by guilt or obligation. From where I stand, however, I see how many of you are doing POP lovingly, generously, and competently. And after you do some more "forgiveness work," you may come to the unexpected recognition that you're actually motivated more often by compassion and love than anything else. At the sunset of their lives, is there anything more you want from your parents than giving them greater comfort and feeling their pride in you? Perhaps the one who gets the most from the giant do-over called POP, may actually be you!

14

WAITING AS OUR PARENTS BECOME FRAILER, WEAKER, SMALLER, AND MAYBE WORSE

MY STORY

My folks had resisted moving from New York so vigorously and I'd had to tolerate long-distance POParenting for so long that, when I finally did find a suitable place and move them close, I'd intended them to remain living there indefinitely—maybe with some additional caregiving support. It was a real comfort to me, knowing that they were finally settled.

When I considered how much harder a second move might be for my progressively aging parents, should that ever occur, I feared that the next move might just claim more from my mother's aging mind and spirit than she had to give. Nor did I anticipate that my father would fare well either if there were unnecessary or repeated residential transitions.

The reason I felt so secure about my parents staying at their assisted-living facility (ALF) through the rest of their days was because, prior to my signing their rental contract, the administrator had verbally agreed to that. I'm a careful listener and pride myself on paying close attention, especially if I'm having an important conversation about my parents' last home.

But as events began to unfold, I found myself uncharacteristically questioning my memory. I recalled being told there might be changes to the ALF contract in the future. But as I remembered it, those changes would be as to pricing. There might be increases to the rent, perhaps annually. It was also stated by the administrator that Lillian and/or Jack might need more help in the future and if so, those fees would be added to the initial charges.

No other changes to the contract we had with the ALF were spelled out. Events such as a corporate buyout of the ALF's ownership, changes in the ALF's policies, and my parents' potential behavioral problems were never mentioned as factors that could lead to termination of their lease. As it turned out, as careful as I'd been and as clear as I thought I was, I hadn't asked about those kinds of contingencies, all of which occurred. Who knew? As I would soon see, not thinking to ask would have serious family consequences.

Upon their arrival new residents were invited to eat a few meals with their more veteran peers at the ALF. It was the facility's way to hospitably offer recently transplanted residents a welcome. I noticed that even that simple a socializing experience seemed stressful for my parents: Jack was uninterested but trying to please Lillian, and Lillian was concerned that she couldn't hold up her end of the conversation.

Jack was no longer predisposed to meeting new people at this point in his life. Although he was pleasant with others, Dad generally preferred my company, Mom's, or his own, over small talk with others. Lillian was still outgoing and enjoyed getting dressed and sitting around talking to others. Perhaps she even sought out other people more because her husband was becoming quieter. At the same time, Mom felt pressure at these meet-and-greet dinners because she had difficulty remembering the names of their mealtime companions and what had been said.

Processing all this new information about the large ALF's physical layout, schedules, people, and procedures would have been taxing for people with far younger brains. I recall feeling grateful that this would be my parents' last move and their final time to learn new schedules and the names of a lot of new residents and staff. I saw that doing simple things was simply becoming harder for both my parents.

We're going to fast-forward this story a couple of years. During those years, my parents settled themselves into their new life and learned what they needed to know to live comfortably in the ALF. I never again saw them make any new real friends but we all developed a comfortable rhythm over time. Mom attended her stretching and yoga classes or bingo activities while Dad did his reading. I visited on certain days during the week and longer on weekends. We all would go together to their many doctor appointments and enjoyed sharing a good medical result when there was one.

The three of us continued to go out for a meal now and again. We'd come back and watch their favorite television shows together or listen to the old oldies on the radio. We reveled in Southern California's sunny winter months. I would chauffeur my parents in my convertible, setting a baseball cap atop Dad's nearly bald head so he wouldn't get sunburned. We'd cruise down to the beaches of Malibu and Oxnard or up the amazingly breathtaking canyons to lookouts where we'd stop and admire the vistas. I'd bring along blankets for Mom who got cool on the afternoon drives. Mom's face beamed with her love of the beauty and Dad smiled contentedly. I remember feeling grateful just to see their faces all shiny and lit up, content knowing I'd done something that brought them such joy.

Some days when we were all together, time almost seemed to slow down, maybe to give us a bit more of itself. It even felt gentle and natural to be with them. During those couple of years when I saw them frequently, my parents' declines almost seemed to slow down. It had even stopped feeling different to have them live close by. In fact, I loved that being so close I was able to see them casually for lunch or spontaneously visit even for a half an hour after they'd eaten dinner.

Eventually my parents did need additional help with their activities of daily living (ADLs) and I added in extra hours of ALF care. The ALF staff did things like help Mom bathe, pick out her clothing and get dressed, and take all her medications correctly. Dad, too, needed some help as time wore on. I must have lulled myself into believing that things would continue on without incident indefinitely, but, of course, that didn't last.

Before long I found myself again dealing with the unexpected. Mom's fall had proven a life-changing event for all three of us. When she was unsuccessful in relearning to walk, the only affordable solution was for Lillian to move to a skilled nursing facility (SNF) that could accommodate her current level of attention. Dad stayed behind at the ALF, not needing skilled nursing and liking it where he knew his way around.

I was devastated for Mom that her cognitive and physical limitations required her to adjust yet another time to another new place. Locating a satisfactory SNF that would accept Lillian had been challenging. After the hospital and the rehab SNF had sent her away for refusing to take water, meds, and food, Mom became categorized as "difficult." This severely limited my choices, and the only SNF I liked that was willing to admit her was far from Dad's ALF, where they'd both lived, and in the next county.

At the SNF, Mom discovered that her new life without mobility would require her to live at the "mercy" of the attendants. Since Mom could no longer come and go of her own volition unless she was in a wheelchair, she needed the staff's help to get to a meal, an activity, or even to bed. Like Blanche DuBois of literary fame, Lillian found herself depending on "the kindness of strangers."

Perhaps she would learn more patience? Unlike other elders who quietly disappear into the background at such times, Mom was determined to stay active and engaged. She tried hard to bend her mind and spirit to that positiveness on the days she could. And on those occasions, I worked with her to encourage her. I think my doing so helped her.

I hated watching my parents live apart. A married couple for more than six decades, their distance felt unnatural to me. I also felt the gravity of what a wrenching trauma it must have been for them, but I was helpless to prevent all the changes and upheaval.

My parents' separation stirred in me the sense that all stable things were beginning to fall apart, and I feared my life would never again feel normal. During the first twenty-five years of their marriage, my parents had never spent as much as a night apart. That had seemed normal to me then. Now, after sixty-something years of togetherness, my mother's conditions and her being labeled "difficult" had necessitated her moving far away from him. To me, it felt like Jack was being left behind.

Neither of my parents talked about these personal matters with me. But Dad didn't seem to feel abandoned. In fact, he acted as if he were enjoying his newly found quiet. Dad loved having the individual time he now was able to have with me, he said. But I noticed that he also seemed quite content to have me leave when my visits were done. Usually he was the one to announce that.

But it was on one of those quiet nights when Dad and I missed Lillian's presence more than we knew. Had she been with him that evening, perhaps she would have reminded Jack to put the necessary thickener into his water as he sat watching *Jeopardy*. But Mom didn't live there any longer, and Dad didn't remember by himself.

Seniors' lungs are extraordinarily vulnerable to a variety of respiratory conditions, including pneumonia, and my parents were no exception. Long after they'd left behind their snowy Northeast winters, my parents continued to suffer from respiratory illnesses and serial hospitalizations. Finally, their doctor suggested they add a thickening powder to their liquids as a precautionary measure. A few tablespoons of this thickener which is fibrous in nature, converts liquids like coffee, water, or juice into a honey-like substance, and prevents the aspirating of liquid into the lungs.

Like many remedies and medicines, thickeners have their downside. I was really touched when Dad revealed: "It's so unsatisfying. I don't ever get to have the refreshing feeling of drinking a glass of water or orange juice. I miss the taste of a real cup of coffee. Mine gets all gooey from thickener."

Between its unattractiveness to him and Dad's short-term memory loss, it made sense that he might forget his thickener without extra prompting from the staff or me. To mitigate his forgetfulness, I'd previously asked the ALF staff to remind Dad to add thickener to his water when they brought him his nightly medications. I'd also asked his waitresses to prompt Dad to add thickener during meals in the dining room. When I'd eat with him at home or take him out, as the good POParent, I'd bring along Dad's thickener—like my good parents used to bring along Cheerios to a restaurant for me, so very long ago.

It wasn't clear what actually happened that fateful night. Maybe because he didn't like it, he accidentally forgot to put thickener in his water. Maybe it was simply that he was ninety-one, tired, and forgetful. And maybe some ALF aide forgot to prompt him. The bottom line was Dad drank enough nonthickened liquid to become ill and require an ambulance. He was taken off to the hospital for yet another battle with pneumonia.

A large corporation had recently purchased Dad's ALF. Apparently, his misfortune was unimportant in relation to their larger corporate interests. They "solved" the problem by promulgating a new rule, a unilateral change in our contract. It stated that any resident in any facility we own who uses thickeners must leave voluntarily immediately or face immediate eviction. As we've been warned in song and in life, in a New York minute, everything can change.

The solution seems to have been invented to prevent future litigation so families could no longer sue the corporation for not more carefully monitoring residents using thickeners. The new rule overturned the ALF's previous promises that, once admitted, my parents need never move again—that they would always be accommodated there. That change to our expectations had been understandable when the ALF wasn't able to provide the level of care Lillian needed, after her fall; but this "no thickener" rule felt brutally unfair.

I tried to review the conversations in my mind that I'd had nearly three years previously with the ALF's administrator, before I'd brought my folks to California. Could I have misheard or misunderstood our agreement about this key point of consistent living for my parents? I even asked myself if I'd heard what I wanted and disregarded the rest. Maybe I'd so hoped this would be their last home that I'd chosen to believe it without thinking through the possible limitations or changes, should the ALF gain new ownership. Hadn't the administrator said there'd be no more new people, places, and things for my parents to have to strain to learn? Apparently, those promises were not as solid as they had appeared. I reminded myself once again to be warier of my POP expectations!

I was in Dad's hospital room when the call came in from the ALF. I fantasized that the heads of the ALF chain had changed their minds; maybe they were offering Dad an apology. At the minimum, perhaps they were calling to recommend another facility where Jack's conditions might be better served. Perhaps they were letting him return from the hospital and stay until I could locate a more suitable facility.

Not really. Jack would never be welcome back at his long-standing home in that ALF. The purpose of the call was to have me accept (telephonic) service of process of Dad's notice of eviction from the ALF. If I didn't, the former administrator, now-corporate employee, warned me: a process server would come to Dad's hospital bedside to serve him his eviction papers. The unbelievable truly had occurred! This all made no sense. Like his wife, Dad also would have to leave his home yet another time and learn a whole new facility, set of aides, a new set of rules and residents—and all because of thickener.

The lawyer in me understood why corporations create these kinds of protocols to protect themselves against future liability, but the daughter in me felt sad and "rejected" for my poor daddy. And the POParent in me was absolutely incensed. Jack had always been a kind man who said "thank you" three times to everyone for everything. After successfully recovering from brain surgery at eighty-nine and all the work that had entailed, now the poor man would have to readjust again to new surroundings—and at ninety-one!

Dad and I were so informed that he could not return home. Of course, I'd done no research to locate him a new facility because, until that phone call came in, I hadn't dreamed we'd ever need one.

Next, I was notified that the hospital planned to discharge him within forty-eight hours. Discharge him to what facility? Release him! Why? Had Dad recovered from the pneumonia? The hospital was forcing Dad's discharge but not because he was healthy, had fully recovered, or had any appropriate facility to go to.

No, the hospital insisted on Dad's discharge because of Medicare's payment rules. These are known as diagnosis-related groups (DRGs), to some they are "the dreaded" DRGs, and they regulate how many days of hospitalization Medicare will pay the hospital for an illness, like pneumonia. Looking for a solution, I wondered if our family could pay privately, outside of Medicare, for Dad to stay on a few additional days while I sorted this all out. But hospitals rarely permit this, and, even had they agreed, his bill would have been astronomical and provided only a temporary fix.

When I'd moved Mom and Dad from New York, I'd spent weeks researching different facilities. When I moved Mom to her SNF, I'd been more pressed but still took the time I needed to find the right place. With Dad, I was given no lead time at all. I found myself becoming outraged. This whole situation felt wrong to me—me the lawyer, the daughter, and the POParent. It felt way wrong.

What happened to the promises, before the corporate purchase, the guarantees my parents could "always" stay at the facility they'd learned to call home? What happened to the notion that sick patients weren't supposed to be dumped out of hospitals without placement in adequate facilities? What happened to the idea that a husband and wife would live together until death did them part? What happened to our institutions treating elders with respect as the heads of our families? What the hell was going on in

this world? Didn't my parents and I have a right to expect anything to go as planned?

I finally calmed down, telling myself that I'd be better off
underreacting. We both would be. My being upset wasn't helping
Dad find a decent place to go. And since I was living under the
dreaded DRG's time clock and, no matter what else I had planned
for those days, I now had to focus on finding Dad's next home. I
neglected taking care of my car, my home, my loved ones, and
myself. I catapulted into high-speed solution mode, locating a
place he'd like. I was clearer this time about his requirements than
when I'd originally searched for the ALF. He liked a facility to be
peaceful and quiet, clean and safe, flexible enough to permit residents who needed thickeners, and local enough to allow his doctors to visit him there. If he could also have a window to look
through and a view of trees, he would be content.

When Lillian had moved to the distant SNF, I hired a young
woman to drive Dad to visit Mom on a regular basis. The visits
took up a good portion of the day: the drive took about two and a
half hours, round trip, and their time together could be another
two, three, or four hours. But even with the help of someone to
drive him to see Mom and occasionally to pick up his cleaning or
do some chores for my parents, POParenting two parents in different locations was becoming a full-time job for me.

I was tired a lot and began to notice a disturbing theme emerging: I never had enough time or resources for everything and
everyone. I wasn't twenty years old either, I had to remind myself.
I accepted that, for a while, I'd have to curtail time with my
friends, limit the number of hours I worked, and be willing to
leave anywhere at a moment's notice for a POParental crisis. I
wondered how long I'd be able to manage this multishift life.

As my parents' disabilities were increasing, my POP responsibilities were expanding. POParenting two advanced seniors who
now had two different sets of doctors, facilities, caregivers, and
needs was beginning to exhaust me. Since Dad needed more care
than he had in the past, I hoped I might be able to reunite my

parents in a single facility, an SNF that could accommodate both their current needs.

I was frustrated by the constant changes and allowed a cloud of depression to briefly descend over me. In that moment, I became filled with my own helplessness and hopelessness. I also foolishly told myself I should be better at predicting these changes. Where would I turn for more help? I began to fear that nothing I'd antici-pated would ever come to pass—except, of course, the certainty of death.

YOUR STORY

There are stages in most POPcycles when it seems that all you can do is enjoy your parents as much as you can while you observe them and their worlds contract. Some of the POP challenge at this time is that there's often little you can actually do to change it.

If you've proceeded this far, you've already chosen this journey; found out what you needed to know to do POP; put various help-ful people, things, and legal documents in place for your folks; and gotten to know their doctors, neighbors, and caregivers. You've seen to it that your parents are being well-fed, clothed, and shel-tered in homes with as much security built in as you and they can collectively tolerate and afford. Since you've already done all that, most of your current POP tasks involve what might be thought of as "maintenance." That is, you go see your parents, check on peo-ple and things that are supposed to be helping them, and change things if and when that becomes necessary.

But with little to actually do, if you're like many POParents, you may begin to worry. You may even obsess on what you've done or not done for your parents by asking yourself: do I have enough precautionary measures in place? Can't I do more? There *are* limits on how much you can do to protect another human being, especially another adult.

Many of your folks, despite having some POP needs, may still be functioning quite well at this point of your POPcycle. Your beloved seniors may still be able to do much for themselves and know a lot, even if all the information isn't immediately available to them. I urge you to follow this piece of advice: never disrespect your aging parents by underestimating them.

Even those diagnosed with fairly advanced dementia may have many parts of their brain still working. Particularly with parents diagnosed with dementia, you may find yourself confused by the extent of their abilities one day, followed by the depth of their disabilities that very evening. It's eerie to see your parent forget your name one day and recall in detail the most embarrassing story from your childhood the next. That same adult you've been tenderly protecting may also turn around and push your emotional buttons or remind you of how poorly—or how well—your family used to function. You and your parents may be aging, but they can still trigger feelings you thought you no longer had.

As you've been observing, aging is idiosyncratic. Each person declines at a different rate. Moreover, when one parent's physical, cognitive, and other limitations far exceed the other's, it can be stressful for everyone involved. The need to take care of a partner, live apart, or be taken care of by your spouse will surely alter the dynamics of any couple. After a long marriage—happy or not so happy—these changes can be devastating and disorienting. Even if your parents have a large age difference, it may still feel shocking. Although predictable that one of your parents might age first, when it actually occurs, it may be wrenching for all of you.

Even when your family is still intact, you may find yourself prematurely grieving the loss of your parents or your family as you used to know it. You may be feeling guilty that you haven't done more when you've really worked hard to be a good POParent. You may be agitated and impatient with many things that ordinarily wouldn't bother you or you may feel depressed.

Although premature grieving is quite common, it can be very troubling. You might not understand some of the intensity of your melancholy, especially since your parents are still very much alive. If any of these are happening to you, it might be particularly helpful at this point to seek out a therapist, spiritual counselor, or a POP Family Coach, someone experienced in these types of matters. Give yourself the gift of a few supportive sessions. Remember, if you're captaining the POP boat, you've got to stay awake and focused, but even the best and strongest captains can benefit from a helping hand.

Sometimes you don't know what to do during the calmer times. You may want to stop their becoming frailer, weaker, smaller and therefore feel frustrated. Then you may decide to do something POP, anything. We've looked at this phenomenon before. Your frustration may result in your making up things to do for your parents. Some of those may be useful. You may ask to have your mom's swallowing retested to see if she can have more fun by being allowed to eat more interesting foods than previously. I did that. Or you might bring in a physical therapist or take your dad to a swimming pool to see if you can lighten his depression with some exercise. I did that too.

Your activities may be fruitful or not, in terms of accomplishing something that your parents truly need. But doing these things may help you, as long as you do no harm by undoing things that are working. Feeling you're doing something useful may be better than sitting around and worrying about your parents, but, as you've seen, it also may have its downside.

At other times you may be feeling very sad, as your parents appear to be failing in front of you and they become less and less "themselves." Your desperation to regain a sense of balance may lead you to fix what *is* working, micromanaging the services and people who are working well. That is not useful.

So, what else might you do that could be? How about this: just sit down and patiently, compassionately, lovingly listen to what's going on for these people who are your parents. As with parenting children, sometimes the most valuable thing we can do with our aging parents is simply be there. Show up for them and then listen to them. Pay attention to what they may feel, want, and need. When you can become quiet within yourself, you can become clearer about what's wanted or needed. You can distinguish whether it's more useful to do another POP action or to give your parents the gift of your attention and interest.

No matter how sad it is, unless they die at a young age, your beloved parents *will* get frailer, smaller, and weaker. And there isn't a lot you can do sometimes except to lovingly wait and watch. Sure, you can go to hospitals and doctors, recreation centers and church with your folks. But if you are looking and listening, you'll see the people you love and looked up to when you were a child are now getting frailer, weaker, and smaller. Often it just plain hurts. But, after all, it's part of the Circle of Life and your being able to reframe your thinking to see it that way may make it more acceptable and less painful.

15

DOING THE ONLY THING LEFT

Comfort-Filling Your Parents

MY STORY

Despite bringing my parents to a warmer climate in the hope of decreasing the number of serious medical events they would have to endure, those situations actually increased in frequency after they became Californians. Their hospitalizations were beginning to occur so often that they felt commonplace but, never ordinary.

Going to the hospital often had proven debilitating for all concerned. Relentlessly these elderly people I loved had battled pneumonias, undergone serious surgeries, endured the even more difficult anesthesia as well as the postsurgical physical and occupation therapies. I saw how all of that had drained my fragile parents, now in their nineties. Being in the hospital with other sick people often made them sicker, exposing Lillian to Methicillin-resistant Staphylococcus aureus (MRSA) and other complications. I, too, became exhausted, as I tried to balance my life while driving incredible distances between home, work, and my parents' respective assisted-living facilities (ALFs), skilled nursing facilities (SNFs), and hospitals.

Aside from a few extraordinary events—like my birth, Dad's hernia operation when I was sixteen, an infamous hurricane in the early 1950s—my parents had been together without interruption. Until Mom moved away permanently to the SNF, each of their hospitalizations and rehabs had required my folks to manage the additional adjustment of living apart from each other. These events emerged as a major life disruption, since, during their six decades of marriage, my parents had arranged it so they spent their days and nights together.

During their early years together, Dad's lupus skin disorder had made him ineligible for the draft. The resulting alternate service he did was local, allowing him to stay living at home with Mom. Even when he had his office in midtown, Dad would often write songs and conduct his music business from home. After I went off to school, Jack gave up his office and shared all his days and nights in the two-bedroom apartment with his wife.

Their hospitalizations demanded other changes from Mom and Dad as well. They had to wrap their minds and aging bodies around spending their days apart and their nights sleeping alone and in beds that were different from those they were used to. It was easy to see how they could have become sleepless or paranoid in the middle of a dark night in a strange bed, drugged, disoriented, not knowing who was coming to help them. This often led to sleep disruptions and/or to extra medications to calm their disorientation.

Being in the hospital also meant being in a whole new environment and relating to the constantly changing staffs there. That became increasingly challenging, and each hospitalization added more to their stress. Jack and Lillian weren't only challenged by their cognitive limitations but also by their vision and hearing, which were no longer all that sharp. Similarly, their postoperative rehabilitation process also required spending additional time away from each other in specialized facilities with their own new staffs to deal with, often uncomfortable beds and consistently novel environments to learn.

All this visibly drained my parents' energies and would have been tough on people years younger and healthier. Their hospitalizations also unsettled my parents' regular routine back at their facilities. Each time it was more difficult to readjust to life back at home. Now that they were in their nineties, even small changes were getting harder for Mom and Dad to accommodate and incorporate. I wasn't getting younger or healthier myself, and, at that point in our POPcycle, I was too often ignoring the very advice I gave others about self-care and knew to be right.

It was becoming clear to me just how exhausted Jack had become when I was figuring out where to place him after his last bout with pneumonia. My father was tired of being sick, sick of hospitals, rehab centers, and the revolving-door ritual these institutionalizations had become. Lying in his last hospital bed, Dad's body looked emaciated. Oddly, being so thin made him look almost like a young boy rather than an old man.

Had I not felt unbearably sad seeing him so vulnerable there, maybe I'd have better appreciated the humor in his point of view.

"Look at these people, Jane. They're unhealthy. They're fat and I don't mean a few pounds overweight but horribly, morbidly obese. Not only that, but they have cigarettes falling out of their pockets. They should know better than to smoke! I'm talking about the doctors here honey, not the patients. How can we trust these people to take care of me when they treat themselves so badly? Get me out of here."

I knew he was right. I'd forgotten that this now-shrunken old man had once been an outspoken health enthusiast, a daily exerciser, and a state champion athlete in his earlier life. Early on when lots of people smoked, Jack proudly told me that he'd never smoked a single cigarette, hoping to discourage my acquiring an unhealthy practice. I smiled, remembering Dad's vision for vibrant health back in the day.

When I went away to college and was no longer under his watchful eye, his contribution to my healthy habits was a weekly delivery of a basket of fruit, arriving fresh every Monday. As a youngster, I'd watched Jack's discipline as he worked out in his bedroom every single morning. No fancy gym, no trainer to keep him on target, Jack just used his good common sense. Now that same man was begging me: "Get me outta here, Jane. I hate the hypocrisy of obesity and smoking by doctors. I'm tired of being here. Plus, it's always freezing in these hospitals. No amount of blankets ever makes me warm enough. Honey, take me home and please never bring me back!"

Notwithstanding the neurosurgeon's earlier disparagement of Jack's brain, Dad revealed he could still articulate his wishes with crystalline clarity. I knew that I should heed his requests. He wanted to be warmer than he'd been in the hospital. Dad understood that he'd been evicted from his original ALF due to their changing rules and could not return there. He also knew that moving would require his adjusting to a new facility, its staff and residents, and different rules.

My Dad stated that he did not want to be placed with Mom in her SNF. Jack explained this in terms of his medical needs, saying that he didn't need the same level of care Lillian did in the SNF. That was accurate, although less true at that point than it had been previously, since he was weaker than ever. I considered that what he really meant by his comment was far different than what he was saying: my now fatigued father didn't want to live with Lillian.

It seemed wiser and kinder to comply with his request rather than try to convince him of something he clearly didn't want in order to simplify my life by having two parents at a single facility. I could see that Dad felt relieved after we'd talked about his not joining Mom at the SNF. He seemed particularly comforted because I'd listened to his hospital-bed requests.

So out I went and found Jack a different, smaller ALF that seemed to provide more supervision than the first had. Fortunately, they had an opening for a male resident when we needed one. This ALF was located a few miles from the old ALF and, significantly, it was near his doctors. If this new ALF fit my POParenting standards for him, Dad could be living there within days and within the deadline that Medicare's diagnosis-related groups (DRGs) had imposed.

I immediately toured the facility and talked with the proprietors, staff, and their residents at some length. It seemed doable. The ALF passed my "smell test"—that is: it didn't smell at all bad and the food smelled good. They also had cameras installed at key locations to keep track of their residents and the attendants. I liked the notion of additional equipment to provide extra eyes on Dad and was pleased to learn that the owners of the facility could watch out for Dad from their homes.

After conducting as thorough a "due diligence" as I had time for, I employed my best intuitive skills to conclude the staff at this ALF would (hopefully) be more careful and attentive to Dad than they'd been at his previous facility. I prayed that the people at the new ALF would monitor him better, since I hated the idea that Jack might forget to put thickener into his coffee and contract another aspiration pneumonia. I was especially fearful of that happening after Dad had been so outspoken about never returning to another hospital.

At this point in the POPcycle, when my parents were able to do few things for themselves and were feeling somewhat powerless, it seemed crucial that, at least in their interchanges with me, they feel as respected and heard as possible. Knowing that I understood their concerns and was heeding their wishes, when I could, seemed more important than ever before.

Dad got into my car at the hospital for this unplanned move with characteristic cool. Early on, he'd decided to be a noncomplainer, teaching it to me this way: "Keep your complaints to yourself, honey. Pay attention and you'll see that nobody really wants to hear them anyway." In his old age, Jack had become a "triple thank-you" giver as I shared earlier. He repetitively expressed his appreciation for almost anything done on his behalf. Dad's quiet, easygoing nature and these frequent expressions of gratitude made him relatively simple to place this time, which contrasted with Mom, who often was accompanied by her challenging attitude and her "record" of previous problems.

Driving Dad to his new ALF, I sensed I was bringing him to his last home, quite literally. The man who had picked out my first home was now graciously allowing me to choose his final one. The new facility was clean, warm—Dad was happy about that—and attractive. Most of the residents displayed more severe aging symptoms and disabilities than their counterparts at Dad's former ALF had. The cameras in the halls, common areas, and at the nursing stations did provide me an odd sense of security, and didn't feel concerned about the possible intrusions on Dad's privacy, since he was my responsibility and I wanted him safe, despite knowing there was no ultimate safety from death.

They gave him a large single room rather than the two-room apartment he and Mom had occupied at their original ALF. I'd negotiated with the owners and gotten Dad more caregiver attention in exchange for less living space. Sunlight filled Dad's room most of his days at his new facility. I arranged his furniture so that he had a separate sitting area, near the entryway, although his guests were few in number. I placed his single bed, where he would spend most of the remaining days, at the far end of the large room, facing the window.

From his bed, Jack could look out onto a beautiful courtyard filled with fruit trees that seemed to be constantly in stages of blooming. I loved to watch my father as he warmed his body with the sun streaming through the window and warmed his spirit with the beauty of the trees and the serenity in his surroundings.

Life went on uneventfully for a while for Dad. I watched him getting used to his new home, and he seemed quietly content. When I'd come to visit, he'd be relishing his peaceful view, reading a newspaper, watching some nighttime television or resting comfortably. I didn't otherwise know how Dad was reacting to all the changes because, like so many men of his generation, he'd never been one to say a lot about his feelings. Nonetheless, when Jack *did* want to make his views known—about not returning to the hospital and not moving into Mom's SNF—he was able to make his point very clearly.

Although he was outgoing and often talkative in his younger days, he'd gotten a bit quieter over time. But now Dad started to become quite "internal" and withdrawn. He was even less forthcoming about himself or his opinions than previously. When he was in the mood for visiting with me, Jack appeared to love talking, but, increasingly, it was he, not busy me, who would be the one to end our visits, claiming fatigue.

Jack was uninterested in a social life with the other people at this latest home and had no need to be entertained by them or the staff. He found no one in the new ALF whom he wished to befriend or particularly even converse with. But that wasn't so very different from his first California residence. Aside from family, Jack preferred to spend his days and nights in a more solitary fashion, a place that he termed "peaceful."

Despite being in a resting mode most of the time and in bed a lot, fatigue seemed to overcome his body, energy, strength, and even his motivation to move. It seemed like his spirit had even become tired, although not necessarily peaceful. Dad seemed to lack purpose for the first time I could remember. It felt like he was off-balance, and not at all himself.

I watched as weariness overtook Jack's mental functioning. As with many writers, my father had always been fascinated with life's details. As he settled into his final home on earth, I witnessed him losing interest in many things. I knew he was slowing down when Dad stopped reading. Books had been a great love for him, a quiet spot in a demanding marriage. Initially, he'd seemed untroubled to find out that he was rereading some books he'd previously borrowed from the ALF's library. Later, he limited his reading choices to shorter pieces, like magazine or newspaper articles. Finally, he stopped reading altogether.

Then, the news and his favorite television shows lost their appeal, and even *Jeopardy*'s mental challenges no longer held his attention. Sometimes I thought he was even losing interest in me. When that happened, I tried to not take it personally. Mostly Dad spoke of wanting to rest, even as he was already lying in his bed.

Observing all these changes still hadn't prepared me for something I didn't really want to see. One afternoon he called me into his room to have the "Talk" he needed me to hear. It wasn't expected. He spoke without hesitation, saying things that I had

difficulty allowing myself to comprehend. So I just listened. "Jane,
you seem to be doing well and you don't really need me anymore."
I resisted telling him I did need him. I wanted my father to feel
vital and strong and for me to be able to lean on him, as I'd done
in my youth. The truth was that he seemed tired all the time and
no longer available for me to lean on. I tried telling myself I
shouldn't need to lean on my father anymore, that I was the
grown-up now. But a part of me wasn't 100 percent sure about
that, the part that still wanted her daddy.

"You know, honey, I'm not going back to the hospital again.
Hospitals are cold places with sick people and I don't see any
reason to return there. I'm done with hospitals. And truthfully
Jane, I feel kind of done with living. I'm always exhausted. I'm
tired of fighting this chronic pneumonia, and I can't remember
the last time I felt well or had any energy. I don't want any more
medication with their gruesome side effects."

He took a long pause and continued on. "I can see that you're
doing fine, honey. More than fine. You're a good girl and you'll be
all right. You've been taking such good care of your Mom as well
as me. I can rest well knowing you'll continue to look out for your
mother. As for me, I'm ready to go. I apologize to you for not
having more energy or sticking around longer. I'm sorry. But can it
be all right if I'm done fighting and allow whatever happens to me
to happen? And if so, what do we do about it?"

I took a breath, realizing I had mostly stopped breathing as
he'd been speaking. My father wanted me to understand that he
felt his living was complete. He was tired of fighting his illnesses,
and, should something lead to his death, he was ready to go and
that would be acceptable.

Dad wasn't hopeless. He wasn't depressed. He wasn't suicidal
as he'd once been back in New York. He wasn't simply insulted
with the hypocritical doctors who didn't live the healthy lives they
espoused nor merely irritated with being forever cold in hospital
beds. He wasn't ashamed that he could no longer do his work or
support others. Jack didn't seem to mind the thought that neither

his daughter nor his wife needed him any longer; if anything, that seemed a relief to him as he faced his current limitations.

My Dad was tired enough to let go of the struggle, willing to release himself. Characteristically, this man of such notable determination considered his death and the process of dying to be his choice. I had just spent the last seven or eight years of my life focused on creating a better life for my folks. I'd tried so hard to make my parents' world—what? "Safe" from death? And now, one of them wanted to walk right into that abyss and give up fighting. A part of me was momentarily confused, I'd say even incensed. I tried reminding myself that Jack's decision wasn't about me. But even though I understood that, I felt profoundly sorry for myself and my "abandonment."

Dad had apologized to that part of me, the one not yet ready to fully accept what he was going through. Of course, he had no reason to apologize for being worn out at nearly ninety-two, not to me or anyone else. But I needed some time to allow the full implications of his decision into my comprehension. I needed to figure out how to manage my emotions and then how to make it happen for Dad with comfort and grace. It seemed so ironic that, just when I was finally becoming a bit adept at being his POParent, I might not be able to do that much longer.

I reminded myself that this was his life. Dad owed me nothing more. He had given me life, his love, an extraordinary education, and the very best of himself. He'd even left me and the world his legacy of music. My more rational self said there was no more that he needed to do for me, not even stay alive.

I breathed in deeply to access my inner calmness. In my most grown-up voice, I heard myself saying, "It isn't your job, Dad, to stay alive in order to amuse or please me. I can't imagine how much I will miss you, but, if you feel ready to go, I will honor that. I'll speak with your doctors and see if you can be put on hospice. And after that, I'll do all I can so that your remaining days and nights are as pain free and peace filled as possible." Somehow, I'd been able to give my father the mature and enlightened POParental response I wanted to offer him.

I drove home and read up about hospice and the requirements of getting Dad into Medicare's hospice program. I learned that Dad would be eligible for hospice services after his physician certified that he was suffering from a terminal condition and unlikely to live longer than six months. Hospice services could be given him in a separate hospice residence or in his ALF. Finally, Jack would not need to return to those cold hospitals nor move again. No, he was home for good.

My next steps involved requesting that Dad's doctor certify him for hospice, which he did, and then choosing one agency from among many that contracted with Medicare to provide him the services allowed under federal regulation. Hospice's palliative care involved rest, water treatments, pain relief for the coughing or discomfort if he wished it, and counseling for any emotional and spiritual concerns.

Once on hospice, Dad would no longer be given treatments to cure any illnesses that might become opportunistic, just treatments that comforted him. Should he get another case of pneumonia, for example, he would not be prescribed antibiotics or other medications to fight it. If Jack wanted to taste his favorite coffee without thickener or eat rich foods again, he could now indulge those cravings.

I was referred to a few good hospices in Dad's neighborhood from other POParents and from my geriatric colleagues. I contacted them, checked out what I could about them online and then went to interview the hospice providers in person, just as I'd earlier done with Mom and Dad's residential facilities.

Hospice workers are generally known in the medical and geriatric communities as unusually kind and caring people. I particularly liked the compassion I saw and heard from the staff at one agency and opted for them. Their people came out to meet with Dad and assess his needs and desires. They offered him warm baths, nutritional services, visits from social workers, conversation with spiritual people, and lots of information. I stepped back to watch how they would do their work—I knew a lot about aging but little about the process of dying.

After that, I went online and ordered every book I could find on "death and . . . *humor*" and asked that they be shipped ASAP. I wanted to find a way to laugh when life was at its most challenging. Or maybe I needed to. But, either way, my instincts said: "this is part of life, too. You might as well enjoy the ride and see the humor." That perspective was something I'd learned from my daddy. I could now honor my mentor by finding and utilizing the funny side of dying.

One evening during hospice when I went by to visit him, I saw a business card on Dad's nightstand. It belonged to the hospice minister who, I learned, had been by to see Dad several times, as it turned out. Jack's parents had not been believers in a religion, and so he had been given no formal religious education. We'd never talked much about his point of view regarding an afterlife. But months before "meeting his Maker," apparently Jack was seeking a spiritual perspective from this hospice minister.

I asked Dad if I might talk to the minister, although I'm unsure exactly why I did that. I think I hoped to somehow reassure myself that Dad was resolving any remaining questions he had, in preparation for his demise. I was pleased when the minister told me they'd talked extensively. It seemed that Jack's comfort was arriving in a variety of palliative packages. I felt very grateful my father had found someone to talk to, maybe as part of his final healing.

Dad had been kind as usual when we talked after he was put on hospice. He wanted to clarify that his decision to go on hospice didn't mean he was "tired of me." Even before his move to California, he'd told me of his excitement to spend more time than we'd had all those years when I'd only visited.

When he became a Californian, Dad delighted in discovering the little things that he felt he could only learn by our spending time together. He'd ask all about me, my work, my ways of being in the world, and how I thought about things. I loved hearing how proud he was of my accomplishments and, more importantly, of how I treated people. Both Dad and I treasured those times together. Now that he was on hospice and our days together were numbered, I tried to make sure to remember it all. I still think about those loving conversations periodically. I bring them out to savor them and they still make my heart sing. But I'm getting ahead of myself.

During hospice Dad seemed to particularly enjoy our just being together quietly until he faded, which was sooner and sooner. It didn't matter whether we talked about anything or not. Sometimes we just held hands as we watched television. I'd already begun working on this book and showed Jack my earliest drafts. As with Mom, I had a hint of trepidation, wondering how he'd respond to the book, to the intrusion it might be on his privacy and also to the notion that I was POParenting him.

I should have known him better and had more faith in him. Dad grinned with fully relished pleasure. Not only did he love the concept of POP, but he also got how much help my work could be. He was joyous about what POP could do for other families. Moreover, he was proud of my blossoming third career. "Imagine, Jane, you're a writer, too! Finally, you're joining the Wolf family business! Your grandmother would have loved your having that potential to influence the world for good, honey!"

Long ago Jack had figured out how to earn his livelihood, as had other Wolf family members, doing work he loved, writing. Several years after Dad left the planet, I got to experience the power of being a writer. It was the morning after Barack Obama was elected president and I was reading his autobiography, *Dreams of My Father*.[1] At that point in the story our new president was chronicling some of the disheartening days he'd had doing community organizing. He had resorted to listening to music for encouragement, and there, on page 91, were the lyrics of Dad's song "I'm a Fool to Want You," which, sung by Billie Holiday, had comforted the future leader of the free world. I swelled with pride.[2]

Like Jack's influence on the young American president, others in our family had been gifted with being able to make a difference in the world through their words. My paternal grandmother as a teenage girl living in Eastern Europe had helped many families escape to the United States from oppressive conditions there. Later, after giving birth to my Dad and his siblings, she'd written a daily column for a political newspaper, advocating for better conditions for workers and the poor. It was virtually unheard of at that time for a woman to be a writer, have her opinions published, and be actively discussed in the community.

Dad's younger brother George had gone in a different writing direction, creating advertising copy and minting phrases that would become America's household names, like the characters in *Mad Men*. My first cousin Dick Wolf, George's son, created, wrote, and produced the *Law and Order* series and more, having emerged as a world-renowned writing icon and almost anyone with a TV can attest to the sway of his written words.

Now, I too might be joining the family business, and it felt right and very good to have Dad welcome me so warmly into it. He called the family's ethos "writing with the intent to make a difference." Up until then, I hadn't seen myself as any part of that or any other tradition. Starting this book had seemed like adding to my psychotherapy and POP Family Coaching practices, not embarking on another career with ancestral roots. But Dad was right, as usual: it was my intention then and has remained my goal to have this book be of service to the world, to make a difference.

Dad and I decided not to tell Mom that he'd gone on hospice. Attempting to explain the concept of hospice to Lillian would have been wasted on her by that time. Nor did we share with her how soon he might pass. Dad and I agreed there'd be no benefit to that, especially since there was no certainty about the time. Having vague and incomprehensible information would likely have caused Mom unnecessary distress, and there seemed little upside, since there was no way she was equipped to understand or prepare herself.

When Lillian's conditions had required her placement in a different geriatric setting from Dad's, many things changed in the dynamic of our threesome. For a couple that had previously spent so little time apart, this separation dramatically altered their relationship. Mom was unable to operate a cell phone and the SNF didn't encourage phoning on their line unless there was an emergency. Hearing on the phone was also a problem for Mom. As a result, in-person visits became my parents' way of communicating with each other, and I was responsible for making the arrangements.

Once they began living separately, my parents needed me to be the connection between them. Mom got carsick on the mountain roads and had greater disabilities, both physically and mentally, so Dad became the logical candidate to be the traveling spouse. That was always the way, except for once at the very end of his life, when I brought Mom to tell him "goodbye."

The frequency and length of their visits together were determined by how much time I could stay, and eventually imposing my time limitations didn't seem fair to do to them. I decided to hire someone to drive him for these visits, which then allowed Jack to dictate how long he'd stay with her. The time they spent together became shorter and shorter, and although Dad would blame his short visits on his driver to Mom, I felt he was purposefully disconnecting from her.

Another consequence of my parents' living apart was that I got to have time with each of them separately. That had rarely occurred since I'd left high school. Back then, Mom had been a bit proprietary, some might say controlling, in insisting that all three of us share as much time together as possible. Even talking on the phone together long distance, Mom aimed for three-way conversations. I missed the intimacy of one-on-one talks with each parent, but these "conference calls" made her less anxious, so Dad and I accommodated her wishes.

My father and I had now gotten into a new routine of talking every day by phone. Now that there was no Lillian on the other phone, it was just the two of us. We would catch up on our respective days. Our end-of-life conversations were filled with sweet words and abundant affection. I'd tell him I loved him. Dad would insist that he loved me more. I would tell him I doubted that possibility. He'd persist, offering proof of his greater love: "after all, I'm older and wiser." It was hard to rebut that evidence.

Until you've actually been through it, it's hard to fathom how debilitating it can be to watch your loved one, especially a parent, become weaker, thinner, and increasingly removed from everything around him. In those concluding months Dad became painfully thin, skinnier every day it seemed. It hurt me to look at his shoulder bones sticking out through his pajama tops. It's still hard to erase the memory of Dad's head sitting on top of a body as thin as any concentration camp survivor.

On some visits I'd bring along my dog to cheer everyone up. I knew from my residency work at the Veterans' Administration how healing a domesticated animal can be, especially for elderly folks. My fourteen-pound rescue dog had a magnetic personality, and I watched how the residents at Dad's facility would perk up when he came on the scene. Although the dog and Jack hadn't developed a significant bond earlier, as Dad's days were dwindling down, my puppy would nuzzle him sweetly with unconditional affection. I'd found another way to provide the comfort care of hospice to my Dad.

By the end, I was making nearly daily visits to Dad just to be around him. I would go by before work to check up on him or after work to feed him, although I wasn't really needed for either. Dad seemed to be eating the ALF's food and reported that he even liked it, but he was still somehow losing weight rapidly.

In spite of his cheerful demeanor and peacefulness, something about his physical essence reminded me of something I'd seen before—in deprived infants. In those cases, it was clinically referred to as a "failure to thrive." I sometimes wondered if Jack had willed himself into that condition after making his hospice decision. Earlier in life he'd seemed capable of creating whatever he'd wanted: a marriage to a woman he adored; a daughter he was proud of (thanks, Dad!); work that he loved and felt meaningful, and a dream home that "Jack built." If that man put his intention into leaving, maybe he was now ready to die by "failing to thrive."

I tried to let that be okay with me if that was what he wanted, but it was hard nonetheless. I kept my focus on Jack and making sure his remaining time on Earth would be special by being as loving as I could and doing things that were full of comfort. I even tried to add some pounds onto him. I'd buy the largest box of Dad's favorite snack, Nilla Wafers, and warm them in water until they reached pudding consistency. Gently I would feed him with a spoon, simultaneously setting my intention to remain calm. Feeding my father, as he'd once fed me, was eerie.

Watching Jack's life clock run down, I wished I could hold back the hands of time. But that wasn't in my power. I was beginning to see that such a desire might be rooted in my own selfishness. Was it I who wasn't ready, maybe? Despite my own pain and grieving the impending loss, I aimed to be unconditionally loving. Sometimes it felt good to know I'd done so much for him and that the rest was out of my hands. At other times I felt horribly frustrated by my lack of control as I watched my childhood hero fade away. I wondered repeatedly whether there wasn't something more I could do but there was really nothing more. The only thing left was to make my father as comfortable as possible and then let him feel peace on his path toward whatever might await him on "the other side."

I waited for some sign to tell me what, if anything, I was to do next. Would Dad develop another case of pneumonia, this time fatal? Would I be strong enough to withhold his medication? As it turns out, I didn't need a sign.

In the very room where he'd told me he was ready to leave, and within six months of the "Talk," Jack's expressed request was fulfilled. There would be no more cold hospital beds, no more adjusting to new facilities with new rules, no more "forgotten" thickener, and no more struggling for Jack Wolf.

THEIR STORY—DAD

I was always very honest with Jane. I thought that was important as a Father. But I'd never told her all my thoughts and feelings. Heck, I hadn't even done that with my wife, my brothers, or anyone else. Men of my generation were never all that comfortable doing the sharing that women seem to thrive on. I'd kept my own counsel quite a bit. That meant I left some things unexpressed and kept a lot to myself. At ninety-one, I wasn't about to start changing all that just because I was living alone or getting old.

Nonetheless, after she'd begun doing all that caring for Lillian and me, I'd really noticed how well Jane was able to listen to me and get what I was saying and feeling, and I appreciated it to no end. I felt that her ability to be fully present and really get what was being said must have served her very well in her legal and psychological counseling. I noticed that, whenever she could, Jane produced whatever I asked for. When I was in the hospital that last time, I was miserable. I was tired of the doctors and endless medication that didn't seem to do any good. I wanted to be warm, get out of there, and go home. Jane listened again and she responded to my requests.

I knew I didn't need to have one or two aides carrying me around from the bed to a chair to the toilet and back, as Lillian did. And I didn't want to go to an SNF, like she had to. What I wanted was to stay in my home where I could rest and have some peace. I know it would have been easier on her to not have the two of us living so far apart, since Jane had taken on the responsibility of visiting and monitoring the care for both of us.

Jane seemed to notice that I was no longer keen to live with Lillian and even our visits together had become pretty short. It was hard because we couldn't really talk anymore, my wife and I. There was so little left we could talk about, most of the time, although occasionally she rallied and I could see the woman I'd married and loved my whole life. She was becoming less and less present. It was as if she wasn't quite there anymore.

Sometimes Lillian was even confused about who I was or why we didn't just go home together. It hurt me to watch her become a shadow of the vibrant woman I'd known. I finally did talk to Jane about some of my feelings, and she was more understanding than I'd expected. I knew if I moved in just to be with Lillian at the SNF, which I didn't need medically, I'd be sad all the time, upset at seeing her as she was but unable to do anything about it.

I was already continually frustrated when I saw how little I could help the woman I loved and had promised to be with 'til death did us part. Her state caused me to hurry off nearly each time I saw her, and I found myself making up excuses to get out of there as soon as I could. All the while, I felt helpless and decidedly unhusbandlike. Again, I tried talking with Jane, and, surprisingly, felt freer for having told her. She listened mostly, and offered a few reassuring remarks, inviting me to assuage my guilt. She said Lillian and I had schooled her well that guilt about the past that couldn't be changed was a waste of energy; now, she wanted to remind me of my teachings.

As a result of all of this, I decided not to spend much time with Lillian in that hospital-like place she lived, and Jane did not fight me at all. My visits became shorter and shorter, as I knew I couldn't peaceably watch the woman I'd so cherished disappear in front of my eyes. I needed to get away and live apart to protect myself from the pain.

Eventually, there came a time when I felt I needed to let her go. She was still alive but only recognizable on the outside. I was still alive but always tired. I wasn't interested in finding another woman or another anything. What I was interested in was finding a way to begin to detach emotionally from Lillian and maybe more. I put up those mental barriers we men do—those compartments—and began thinking of myself as a widower, not a husband. I continued to visit Lillian and stayed as long as I could, but mostly my sweetheart had already gone. And I was allowing that to be all right. I let these changes process through my system, and then I looked around me. My daughter was doing fine. My wife was beyond my grasp and effectively gone. I was tired. Maybe I wasn't much needed here anymore.

YOUR STORY

Hospice is an alternative type of health care offered in the United States under the Medicare program to eligible people, including

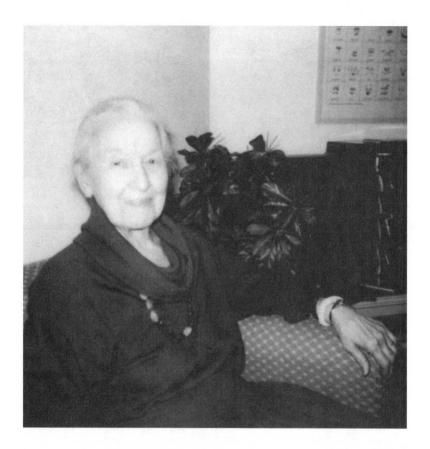

Figure 15.1. **Mom still elegant at eighty-nine**

perhaps your parents. The requirements include having a diagnosis of a terminal illness with an expectation of no more than six months to live. Hospice care focuses on offering the palliation or relief of the person's symptoms, rather than on curing any underlying disease.

Some think of hospice as being limited to pain relief or that it has to be provided in an institution, but neither of those is true. Since the symptoms your parents may be experiencing during this time in their POPcycle might be physical, emotional, spiritual, and even social in nature, hospice offers relief from all of these. The

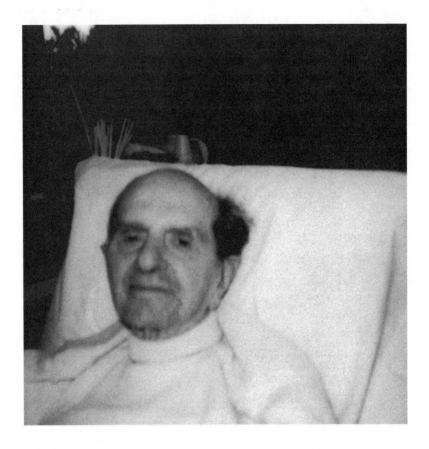

Figure 15.2.   Dad, eighty-nine, recovering from brain surgery and learning to walk again

services provided by hospice agencies can be given in your parents' own home, their residential facility, or in a specially designated hospice facility.

The idea of hospice care has been around for many centuries, long before there was Medicare or a United States of America, but hospice care in twenty-first-century America is designed to permit patients like your mom and dad to be kept as comfortable as possible without having to undergo more rigorous treatments aimed at curing their illnesses.

Once your parents request to be put on hospice, meet the qualifications, and get certified by a physician, you and your parents can choose a particular hospice agency from a list of such agencies that have a contractual relationship with Medicare. The agency will provide your parents the following services, and Medicare will pay the costs in all or nearly all the following categories: [3]

- Doctor services
- Nursing care
- Medical equipment (such as wheelchairs or walkers)
- Medical supplies (such as bandages and catheters)
- Drugs for symptom control and pain relief
- Short-term care in a hospital
- Home health aide and homemaker services including respite care for caregivers
- Physical and occupational therapy
- Speech therapy
- Social worker services
- Dietary counseling
- Spiritual and other counseling for your parents and family

Your parents' out-of-pocket charges will be very limited, if any. While on hospice, your parents are entitled to have a person help care for them. That person can be a family member. Medicare even offers respite care to your parents' designated helper and, during that time, a supplemental caregiver is provided to them.

The decision to go on hospice will be made by your POP family and your parents, if they are competent to do so, in conjunction with your parents' physician. You needn't be concerned that being on hospice means your parents will be medically neglected or overlooked. Quite the opposite, the hospice staff will provide medical and nonmedical services for your parents, just different types of services than traditional Western medicine. They will receive comfort care without the expectation of recovery. It may be very calming, relieving your parents of burdens you didn't even imagine they were bearing.

Hospice care is provided in increments of time. Your parent can receive it for as long as the doctor certifies that less than six months probably remain for the patient's life. If the patient lives longer than six months, hospice care will be continued, provided the doctor recertifies it. Under current Medicare regulations, your parents are eligible to get hospice care for two ninety-day periods, followed by an unlimited number of sixty-day periods.

Hospice certification is not an irreversible one-way street. That is, should your parent unexpectedly begin to recover from whatever illness the doctor had thought terminal or, simply, if your Mom gets a change of heart, a decision can always be reversed. She can go off hospice care at any time and fight that illness.

After counseling families who had embraced hospice when the time was right, I came to truly appreciate the many benefits POP families can derive from hospice care. In addition to granting your aging and sick folks some physical and spiritual comfort, this choice can benefit them and the POParents, psychologically as well. Making the hospice decision has restored a sense of control to many a senior parent, newly confident because they feel more in charge of their treatment and their remaining time. That may be particularly true for seniors if they've felt at all disempowered by the POPcycle or if their dealings with Medicare, the health system, or insurance sectors have left them feeling somewhat impotent.

Your parents may be oddly relieved that they'll no longer have to "perform" medically. Surviving difficult chemotherapy treatments or putting up with painful procedures may just require more of your aging relatives than they feel they have, at their advanced age. If your parent tells you: "I've had enough" or "I want to be at peace: let us talk to the priest," you need to get that.

Perhaps you will need to acknowledge your own mixed feelings in the decision. You may have complicated beliefs about "putting your parents on hospice." To become more comfortable with this complicated choice, this would be a good time to employ the POParenting tool of reframing what you've learned in order to think differently and more productively. Notice that you are actually being the best parent and friend your father could want by listening to his request for no more cold hospitals or medicines with their intrusive effects.

Your parent's decision to go on hospice can trigger many different emotional reactions. You may feel frustrated, relieved, and upset that they will soon leave you all at the same time. You may feel disappointed, since you invested so much into POParenting them for years and now they're just giving up. If you listen carefully, you may also discover that what your parent wants most is what he's going to get from hospice care—peacefulness, comfort, eating what he wants, and resting. Letting your dying parent know you hear him and respect him is wise POParenting, at this stage as at others. It is also kind. It probably took your parent a whole lot of thinking and courage to have the "Talk" with you.

Sometimes your parent's physician may initiate the conversation about hospice with you and your siblings or with your parent directly. Or you might ask the doctor to raise the issue with your mom or dad, should it be on your mind. Had it been left up to me, I probably would have continued along as we'd been doing, with Dad going in and out of cold hospital rooms more and more often until his eventual demise. But by his raising the topic of hospice, Dad actually made it easier for me to hear him and then to empathically contemplate what this magnificent, creative, loving, and generous man's life had become. Ever my teacher, he remained so until the end.

When your parent's discomfort or prognosis warrants it, you or your sibling may be the one who needs the courage to bring up hospice. That's especially true if your mom or dad can't. If that falls to you, one suggestion is this. Try talking to your parent about what he'd want for you if these were your sunset days and you were actually in his shoes and he in yours. He is still your parent and that question's odd reversal might provoke some useful communications, including about hospice. It's likely you will also wish to inform him of what you've learned about its many benefits and possibly disabuse him of the assumption that he'd need to leave home.

When conversations about hospice are going on, you may find you're feeling increasingly anxious. You may be concerned about how little time is left in your parents' lives or become worried—about how little time you have left with them, your own death, or how to process their upcoming departures. You may even be dismayed by your parent's' end-of-life choice. If that's the case for you, try to keep in mind, it's *you* who has this problem—your parent is fine with the choices. As a loving POParent, it's unnecessary and maybe even unkind to lay these feelings on your parent, especially once he or she has made the hospice decision.

Perhaps you still have unresolved issues with your parents and doubt those can be resolved in only six months. Consulting a qualified professional therapist or POP Family Coach, even for a few sessions at this particular time, has helped many, and it's likely to help you. You will want to release the feelings that seem to result in negativity or conflict and doing some work on yourself can provide renewed energy and better ways to help you complete the POPcycle with grace. Giving yourself some short-term help during challenging points in your POPcycle, like this one, often produces unexpectedly useful and profound results. On the other hand, not resolving your concerns may further stretch already-strained relations between you and your parents.

Please note that I didn't say you needed to involve your aging parents in your own resolution process. If you still feel the need to resolve your issues directly with your parent(s), before confronting them, stop. Ask yourself this: "Do my mom and dad really *need* to know now how I feel about something that may have happened fifty years ago?" Probably not. "Is there anything my parents could do that would change the past?" If answering those doesn't dissuade you from raising unnecessary historical material with people who may not recall what they ate for breakfast, ask yourself: "How would discussing my issues help my mom or dad?"

Frankly, your parents have bigger things to deal with at this time than your difficulties with the long-ago past. You would be wise to find a different person to air your old hurts or missed opportunities to than your mom and dad. Given the limited time you have left with them, wouldn't the time be better spent focusing on joy that is currently available than sadness from the past?

If you and your siblings are upset with your parents' imminent death or other end-of-life choices, that lack of acceptance may engender a problem of its own. During hospice what your parent needs most is comfort in its various physical, psychological, and spiritual forms. That means this time is as stress free as possible. Conflicts between you, your siblings, and others on your TEAM POP may bring much stress to your parents, and that helps no one. You must be wary to see that dissent doesn't happen especially in front of your parents and to do your best to get along.

For example, if your mother chooses hospice, your POP job is to acquiesce and align those on TEAM POP to be on the same page, helping your beloved, ailing mother toward a serene transition. As you become more comfortable with the choice and more accepting of your mom's decision, she *will* be able to rest better. If going on hospice or working with a particular hospice agency feels right to your mother, it could be the very best choice. After all, it *is* her life.

In a very helpful book called *Companioning the Dying: A Soulful Guide for Counselors and Caregivers* the authors report that the dying are most often and best comforted by those unafraid to stand with them and their decisions without judgment, advice, or expectation. As they move through this extraordinary passage, your parents want your companionship in this courageous way. Even in their final journey, it seems your parents still long to be connected to you and derive comfort from that connection. It may be a small consolation to you that the only thing left to do is to become as calm and compassionate as you can, but that may be the best way to support your parents at this time.

But then again, maybe not. It's also possible there may still be some important or cutting-edge interventions you can try in your parents' situations that I was unable to do in mine. For example, my instincts about Jack's failure to thrive led me to do further research after his passing about what was then a relatively new syndrome. Adult failure to thrive (AFTT) may be caused by multiple chronic conditions and/or the losses associated with limited and decreased functioning. Your mom and dad may be experiencing one or all four AFTT syndromes that are predictors of adverse outcomes: impaired physical functioning, malnutrition, depression, and cognitive impairment. If your senior parents are showing significant decline and weight loss and their physicians are unable to attribute it to any medical condition, ask them to check for AFTT. Many interventions by the medical and hospice communities have resulted in positive changes and a lifting of the AFTT symptoms. It's certainly worth your inquiring.

16

LETTING GO OF THE BELOVED PARENTS WE'VE PARENTED

MY STORY

I put off this chapter until I'd written all the others. It was simply too tough to have to relive my last goodbyes, first to Dad and then to Mom. When people you love have had lives as long and fulfilling as my parents had, for the most part, it's not necessarily sadness those of us left behind are feeling.

For me, it was subtle and not the same as sadness. It was as if I became very conscious of their "nonpresence" on the planet. Even today I sometimes find myself saying: "If he were here, Dad might say. . . ." And just talking about them and remembering them out loud eases the residual eeriness of my parents' relentless "nonpresence."

I remember when I first heard about death. My folks had a family friend who was a legendary film actor named John Garfield. His kids and I used to play together. I was about to turn five and he was barely thirty-nine. One day he had a heart attack, and the next he was gone. I recall thinking: "How odd is that? Our friend Julie (his real name, not the screen name given him by Warner Bros.) woke up dead on Wednesday. I hope it didn't hurt him." I wondered how David and Julie are bearing up without their dad? "What is it like to wake up being dead?" I thought.

As I took in the larger meaning of this one man's death and saw how it affected his family and mine too, I slowly recognized that, someday, all of us would die. My parents would die and leave me too, just as Julie and David's dad had left them. Later I would learn that the man whose death I pondered for months had the largest funeral attendance for any actor since Rudolph Valentino had passed. No one gets out alive. Not even me! For many years thereafter, a part of me lived disquieted by the inevitability of that fact. I have made some peace with it, over these years and POP supported that acceptance.

Starting with my college years, when I'd moved away from my folks, each time I'd part from them after a visit, I'd think that this might be the last time we'd all be together, and, for a while I would continue "obsessing" about it. I define obsessing as rethinking the same thought without resolution, as if I were on a continuous mental treadmill. Reminding myself of the fragility of my family by replaying that dreaded thought sapped me of energy and generated depressing feelings. I realized I was putting myself through a lot of unnecessary angst, and it did absolutely no good for anyone.

So, I worked long and hard to devise tools—which I've been sharing with you—to help me interrupt the anxiety I was generating with such thinking. I taught myself to avoid obsessing over these thoughts by creating a series of steps I could take to prevent myself from staying caught in that one destructive thought. After figuring out the technique, I still needed to practice it by engaging with the process over and again. As a result of doing that, I was freed up to feel calmer and calmer. Eventually, if that thought showed up at our departures, its recurrence did not trouble me much, if at all.

My simple four-step process began with simply allowing myself to notice myself having that thought again, the one about "our last time," without any judgment about its happening, almost like I was watching the thought go by. Next, I saw that thought as merely one among tens of thousands I knew myself to be having every day, subtly diminishing this particular thought's significance. Third, I interpreted the thought for what it was—a mere symbol of my feeling alone or abandoned, not the reality of that happening to me, again minimizing its impact. Last, I interrupted that isolative, sad interpretation with a more positive one, by reminding myself: my fears—symbolic or not—were ideas I'd made up. My old idea had no basis in reality, as neither Jack, Lillian, nor I had any imminent plans on dying, and their love for me could never be lost.

Instead of something to fear, I'd ask: what was something I could be grateful for in this very moment? The answers my mind found to that inquiry were numerous and included my gratitude for the time I had left with my parents. By replacing my worry and other upsetting thoughts with thankfulness, I came into the present and watched my apprehensions about the future begin to fade. It felt as if I were refreshing myself with the flow of gratitude, like the cool spray of a sea breeze on a relentlessly humid day.

When I remembered to do that four-step process, it became much harder to be pulled down emotionally by my own nagging, negative thoughts. To be fair, though, however predictable it was, I found it hardest to remember to use the process in the days immediately preceding my parents' passings. Like most people, I'd often forget my tried-and-true tools when stressed, which, of course, was when I could have used them the most.

I thought I would more often "remember" to get relief if I could narrow it down to three simple steps: breathe in and out a few times; come completely into the present; feel gratitude! Couldn't be easier. Nevertheless, some days even doing that was "hard work." That seemed particularly true when I was feeling sorry for myself, so I'd "try harder" to locate the wellspring of gratitude I knew I had down in me somewhere.

But how to find it? I often employed gratitude lists, mentally checking off everything for which I felt grateful. I'd start with myself. I was alive and breathing; I could see, feel, smell, touch, and taste. My mind was still sharp. I had the capacity to create this list and even remember what I was grateful for. I was healthy (knock on wood!) and had a great support system of people who wanted to share themselves. I had a family who dearly loved me. And, most of all, I was thankful I could be there for Mom and Dad in their final days.

As I got on a roll inventorying my gratitude, a shift would occur inside me. I'd begin to warm to how much goodness there was around me and even feel more protected. I could sense my gratitude expanding into peacefulness. These tools absolutely resulted in my becoming a much more appreciative daughter and, in turn, a happier woman.

Another way I learned to "comfort myself" was by finding a spiritual philosophy that offered me the optimism I wanted to embrace. Through that, I was able to see our human form as one part of a larger and ongoing divine experience and to realize that we might lose our physical connections but never our attachment through love. I'd also been educated to the remarkable powers of the human brain and body to send and receive communications of love, even at great distances. Intervening in Jack's suicide attempts years before was one of many such times I'd witnessed that "miraculous" kind of knowing at a distance about people I loved.

So, at this juncture of our POPcycle, when the time came for the three of us to have our last time all together, I'd done enough work on myself to be able to be less concerned with my own loss to concentrate more fully on my parents and their losses. Through practicing these techniques of detaching from fearful thoughts and invoking gratitude, and through my years of POParenting, I could see I'd expanded my compassion and even lost some of my self-centeredness.

Dad was far more cogent and also verbal about it than Mom, but I was interested and pleased to note that they both perceived their imminent demises to be less about tragedy or loss than about relief from some of the burdens of being mortal. Shakespeare's Hamlet spoke of it in his famous "To be or not to be" soliloquy as follows: "To die: to sleep, no more; and by a sleep, to say we end the heartache and the thousand natural shocks the flesh is heir to."

In the Western world, we have an almost knee-jerk reaction to hearing of someone's death. Even without knowing any details, we call it a "tragedy"! But maybe that's not so. Perhaps if your highest goals involve living a full life, contributing what you have to give, being a loving human, and feeling loved, once you've accomplished these, your death need not be considered "tragic." Perhaps a better description would be "fulfilled." I prefer to consider that the death of such a person is an opportunity for a glorious tribute, an outpouring of expressed appreciation and positive reflections. It seemed my parents did, too.

After months of obvious decline, Dad truly appeared to have little time remaining and little energy left. When I talked with the hospice staff, they agreed his energy was at an all-time low and his attention span was similarly waning. The number of hours he was sleeping had been growing markedly. They said that was another clue that, soon, he'd be at his end. His waning interest in food, other people, activities, or television was extending to everything else. I watched my daddy as he was taking the final exit ramp from life's highway.

I felt strongly that my parents should be given a thorough opportunity to say their goodbyes to each other. Given her limited cognitive state and our concern for her emotional stress, we'd never explained to Mom that Dad was in hospice or the severity of his conditions. Nonetheless, I felt I owed it to them, as individuals and as a couple, to share some last private moments together. It no longer mattered, as it had earlier, how much each of them would exactly understand about what was occurring. I didn't concern myself that Mom might be confused or Dad might want peace and quiet. I just went on instinct that they were entitled to a fond and formal farewell.

I picked Mom up early in the morning from her skilled nursing facility (SNF). During the long drive to Ventura County, I tried to prepare her by explaining that Dad might seem very poorly to her, much weakened compared to how he'd been when he'd last visited. It was her first visit to Dad in this assisted-living facility (ALF) and Lillian was curious about where he was living. When we entered his room, Mom was clearly delighted to see her husband again, as she always was cheered by his presence in these years. But she was clearly confused and distressed by Dad's weakness, skinny body, and low energy.

I respectfully left the lovers who'd created me to savor their final embraces and private words. I'll never know what they said there that day or how much either was able to understand about the implications of the visit. While they were having their private time in Dad's room, I sat in the corridor and tried to envision what this moment might feel like for each of my parents.

Did Mom really get that she was going to outlive the man she had loved for as long as she could recall? Did she fear she couldn't manage without him? Was she angry with Dad for "leaving" her by dying or "abandoning" her by not moving into her SNF?

How about Dad? Did he still feel that choosing hospice was best for him and them? Did he feel upset for "abandoning" the woman he'd pledged to take care of? Was Jack relieved to be free from the challenges of Mom, her illnesses, and his inability to fix these, as well as to be free from the burdens of a physical body? Had they each been preparing themselves for this goodbye for decades?

I started imagining what this moment would be like if it were I, instead of Mom saying goodbye to the man who'd been my family and partner for over six decades: I huddled under a cozy blanket in a wheelchair, he seated next to me, his hand in mine. Whereas once we'd been new to each other, now I am gazing at a face more familiar than my own. Contemplating being about to have our final embrace for all of eternity, I see memories come flooding back: when we'd wed, raised our child, run our music business, and built our home. We'd journeyed thousands of days and nights together, having left behind the places where we'd grown up, our parents and siblings and friends all buried back there. We'd come this far to where we are being cared for by the daughter we'd made and loved together since her birth. I compare those times with him with my days ahead, knowing that I'll be alone. I am holding my gaze on the face of my beloved, a face I'd wiped tears from when we'd shared family losses, a face I'd seen laughter and wisdom etch lines into over the course of a lifetime together. I kiss those lines around my lover's lips and eyes for the last time and try to hold them in my memory bank for all the times ahead when I'll need to remember those golden days. I catch a glimpse of my husband's tired, now skinny arms, the same arms I'd felt safe and loved in for so long. His were the arms I'd reached out to, held onto, and known peace in. Soon I'll need to release those precious arms forever, have only one last hug, an eternal good-night kiss, perhaps a parting laugh or a shared song together.

I had to stop my fantasizing there; my tears were welling up and flowing down my face. To me, my parents' finally separating was incomprehensible in its sadness. It was more than I wanted to grasp. And if all that weren't challenging enough, my thoughts then went to myself. How would the imminent end of our little family alter my life? The Wolf threesome we'd been in many ways since my childhood was coming to a close. Soon we'd be a trio no more.

Most of my thoughts that day were over the top, but I gave myself permission to go there. The day I'd "dreaded" for so many years, the day my family was together for its last time, was a good enough excuse for some melancholic musings. So, I let myself get into the feelings deeply and let them touch my soul.

Then came that fateful Monday in November. Before going to my office in the early morning, I drove over to check on Dad. As I entered the building, several hospice staffers approached me. "It's likely that today's the day," they stated quietly. For a minute I was confused, stopped in my tracks. What did that mean? How did they know? What was I supposed to do next? How was I to react to such information? I took some very deep, remarkably cleansing POParental breaths. And then I knew that I already understood whatever I'd need to know at that moment. I had long awaited it and, now, it was here. I was oddly clear.

My first step was to call my nearest and dearest and let them know the information I'd just gotten about Dad's status. I asked them to come and support me and Dad, as well as bear witness to his imminent passage. I wanted him to have only a beautiful, serene gathering of four loved ones, none of whom would bring in drama and turn Dad's event into being "all about them."

Then I saw to it that all my patients and other appointments for the day were canceled. Having done that, I was now clear of other obligations and free to concentrate on what would be needed of me over at Dad's, whatever that might be, one final time.

Next, I decided I'd feel most comfortable, in this totally uncomfortable situation, were I to return home and change from my professional attire into more "comfortable" clothes. While there, I could pick up whatever "supplies" might feel appropriate for the occasion of Dad's passing. At home I looked for a loose-fitting outfit; specifically, I wanted to put on a fabric that felt good next to my skin. I chose nothing black—too negatively mournful. I looked around for what else might provide me comfort of any kind and grabbed my worn copy of Ernest Holmes's *The Science of Mind*.[1] This wonderful book had served me well as a source of exquisite enrichment for decades. Finally, looking around, I scooped up my dog and brought him along for the emotional comfort he would hopefully provide Dad, and me, as well.

It was with a very full heart that I drove back to Dad's ALF for a second time that morning. This time I knew I was going to say goodbye to my father. Walking into his room, I knew immediately I should move with almost reverential grace and peacefulness. It was eerily still, almost as if his bedroom had transmuted into a sacred space where silence and order were natural and fitting. Dad was pretty much as he'd been earlier, resting fairly peacefully, almost without consciousness. He never became more alert or active in any way.

I opened the blinds, letting in the day's last sunlight for Jack to see or, at least feel, the late autumn warmth. I checked to see if his eyes strained or even moved with the brightness of this new light, but they did not. All was still. I paced a bit around his room, straightening out a few things to create more order. I thought of how odd but intuitively fitting it was to want to impose external order at precisely the moment I felt so internally disoriented. I tried to stay busy, occupied, and useful in some way. Whether or not any of that was constructive, at least I was doing no harm.

Staying busy felt somehow more purposeful than standing still. It was old programming, but productivity felt comforting and anything comforting just then was okay with me. I considered new ways I might bring Dad the "palliative care" he'd requested when he originally asked to go on hospice as I placed the little dog I loved gently next to the father I loved. My hope was that, as his soft canine fur pressed up next to my Father, his rhythmic breathing would provide Dad ease in its regularity. I even wondered if, as Dad was exiting the planet, this contact would remind him of when he'd entered it, breathing right up next to another body.

Another palliative effort I tried was tuning Dad's radio to the station that played the "The Music of Your Life" format. For a moment, Rosemary Clooney was alive again, singing her hits and working with Dad in their early days. I hoped that a disk jockey might choose to spin a Jack Wolf song as his last sun began to settle in the west. I didn't hear any of Dad's compositions that afternoon.

But listening to their selections as the day slowly faded into evening reminded me of the music of my childhood, when my daddy had become my all-time favorite songwriter. He'd come home from Tin Pan Alley and the Brill Building brimming with tales of "peddling his songs," as he called it. These were the same songs I'd been asked to write down when he'd originally thought them up at his favorite muse site, the bathtub. He'd call out from behind the shower curtain: "Lillian or Jane! Come here! Bring a pen and pad!" I'd scurry in, trying to be there first to write down the lyrics.

Later on, after the lyric writing/bath stage, Jack would choose the best composer from among his favorites to work on a particular piece. Thereafter he might contact his early partner, Burt Bacharach, who primarily wrote with Hal David, or Joe Darion, the composer of the beautiful "Man of La Mancha"; Bugs Bower, who also wrote "Itsy Bitsy Teeny Weeny Yellow Polka Dot Bikini"; or Joel Herron, with whom Jack wrote his hauntingly beautiful standard "I'm a Fool to Want to Want You." Then he and the other writer would collaborate and make their respective parts into a song.

Next Dad would go into the studio to create a demo record with simple vocal and instruments to play for prospective record companies, recording artists, and others, showing how the song would ultimately sound. Then he'd "shop the demo" and, "miraculously," out would come—fabulous 45 RPMs (funny-looking records with little holes in the middle) and 33 1/3 LPs [larger, long-play] vinyl records)!

The sound of the familiar old tunes on the radio felt reassuring to me. Thanks to him, I knew almost all of them. And though I'll never know this, I believed the old favorites comforted Jack as well. After listening for a while, I joined in to sing along. It just seemed like the right thing to do. I sang with all my soul to my departing dad, trying to reach into his heart with the love in my voice. Neither my off-key vocalizing nor anything else disturbed Jack's reverie that day.

He was in his own world. I like to believe he heard the music and knew my loving intentions, but even if Frank Sinatra himself had come back to croon for Dad, I'm not sure he'd have noticed. Hours passed as the November dusk turned to evening. But in Dad's room, a part of me wanted time to stand still. My breathing seemed to have slowed down to a pace similar to his. I walked outside for a few minutes for a breath of new air. That was actually helpful, although a part of me didn't want to leave his side for even a moment.

Then I remembered I'd brought along *The Science of Mind*. When I picked up the large book and let it fall open at random, I not-so-secretly intended it to open up on some unexpected spiritual support. When I read the passage I'd "accidentally" opened to, I almost fell off my chair. I smiled, believing that the universe was, even this afternoon, on my side. It seemed like Dr. Holmes had written this for me and for this very occasion.

> What about Death? *The Science of Mind* teaches the eternality of life. It accepts that our physical bodies operate within a natural cycle of birth and death. However, even though we may have a body, we are not just our body. What we really are is the Life that animates our body, and that Life is infinite and immortal. As we become increasing identified with our divine and eternal nature, our underlying fear of death begins to dissolve and our experience of life become more joyous.[2]

At a point of such sadness and despair this random reading arrived like amazing grace, redefining death as I had been thinking about it. My faith was reaffirmed as a warm blanket symbolically wrapped itself around the parts of me that had been cold.

The "invitees" I'd asked to Dad's room included my adopted brother, Rick—the person on the planet who'd known me the longest aside from my parents—and his girlfriend at that time. She was a talented and respected healing professional whose powerful work included "helping people ease their path off the planet." I remarked at the synchronicity of events, for, although they lived up the coast, she and Rick "just happened" to be staying with me in Southern California on that day. She generously offered to help Dad and, although I had no idea what her work really entailed, I anticipated no harm and gratefully consented.

I watched as she prayed and made various gestures over parts of his body. She occasionally asked me questions to assist her mysterious process. Beginning at his feet and moving upward I saw Jack's body noticeably soften beneath the motions she was making. She was working over Dad's chest and heart region for a while and finally asked: "How long has Jack been apart from his wife?" Although she knew nothing of my parents' history, she stated matter-of-factly that Dad was still "working through that separation." I was awed by her suggestion that Dad might still be resolving his issues as close to his earthly transition as this was.

I have no proof that her healing movements, words or prayers helped Dad in any way. Nonetheless, I choose to believe that her appearing on my doorstep on the day of Dad's transition was a remarkable gift for Jack as well as for me.

I've been fortunate enough never to have been at war or in a fire, earthquake, or other disaster where someone died right next to me. Until that day I'd never seen the passage of a human life, someone taking in and exhaling his last breaths. It felt like an honor to be permitted to attend such a special moment in the life of any other person, especially in the sacred space of your beloved parent's last breath. As sad as I'd felt previously, I was very conscious of feeling fortunate to be present. I took a deep breath to center myself and then a few more breaths as I aimed to become fully present to what was about to occur.

I found a place to sit on the narrow bed where his emaciated body lay peacefully. I reached out and held his hand in mine. I lifted it to my lips and smelled my father's skin as I kissed his frail hand. I hoped the warmth of my touch would please him and that my affection would reassure him. I watched the rising and falling of Dad's chest, his breathing had become nearly imperceptible now. It contrasted with my dog's strong, regular breathing alongside of him. Imperceptibly, my beloved father's breathing quietly stopped. I wasn't sure when it happened. There was no obvious body wriggling, no sign of pain, and no evidence of a struggle! Dad had been released from his body's constrictions and limitations.

Afterward, Rick's girlfriend related what she'd seen: Dad's spirit lifted up from where his body was still lying on the bed and, just before it ascended toward the sky, it came from behind and wrapped itself around me in a hug. I took delight in that possibility, one of those ideas we're offered that can give us joy, should we choose to accept it. And in the dark of that unforgettable November night, I believed her. What I'd seen and what was clear to me was that Dad, as I knew him, was gone. There was now only a body that remained behind with us in the room and this felt noticeably different than earlier in the day when Dad lay there nearly comatose. Now, his essence was gone. Jack Wolf belonged to the ages, and thereafter, I had only my memories of him.

The next morning when I drove down to tell Mom about Dad's transition, I was clearly withdrawn and sad. She sensed immediately something was wrong. When I explained the reason for my melancholic state, she became something akin to giddy, seemingly intent on amusing me out of my sadness. Maybe it was Mom's way of comforting me or her grief or just someone at her stage of cognitive decline reacting in a way we'd say was "inappropriate."

In the midst of all this, Mom showed me a new white-haired resident at her facility that she found attractive. With an uncanny use of her verbal skills, she told me: "What a great haircut that handsome man has! I'm sure he also uses expensive hair products. He must be well-heeled." What? I was dismayed at Mom's apparent detachment from what had just happened to us all: to her husband, her—our—threesome, and yes, to me. Even understanding her conditions, I momentarily allowed myself hurt feelings.

Although Lillian seemed unable to fully comprehend that her husband had passed away, it occurred to me later that maybe I'd been wrong about that. I considered how Lillian's "pre–women's liberation" mind might be interpreting the events from within her world. Maybe she did understand that her husband was gone and that his passing affected her status: moving from "married" to "widowed" at age ninety-two. Mom's generation, as those before her, was taught a woman needed a man to take care of her. Maybe her survival skills had kicked in, and Lillian was already "moving along" to scout for decent candidates for her next husband? It seemed so out of place, as I was just beginning to mourn the loss of her last one.

I was always intrigued when "my old Mom," would peek out through the veil of her dementia and other illnesses to have a more lucid awareness of herself and others around her, however temporary that was. Mom's medical situation was complicated. During her advanced years, her body that had so resiliently withstood diseases earlier, developed a series of debilitating pneumonias and a deep disturbing recurring cough.

When the cough reappeared, it would inevitably lead to another course of antibiotics. Antibiotics are "wonder" drugs in many instances but their usage is controversial because they can severely weaken some patients, including many elderly patients. I hated that she was prescribed these powerful medications so readily, since they killed off not only the bad bacteria but also her good ones. However, I also understood that, unless they treated her with these drugs, she probably would not survive.

Every few months usually late into the night, it seemed, I would get a call from her SNF. "Lillian had been feeling poorly." or "Lillian was running a fever," or most often, "Lillian's cough has just gotten too intense." California law requires facilities to contact the next of kin to advise them when a resident is taken to the Emergency Room. Almost always the hospital would admit Mom. I'd go over and usually leave her as I found her, sleeping soundly and connected up to a series of monitoring machines. When she was awakened, Mom would often be confused but, seeing me whether in those foreign settings or at her home, always brought a smile to her face.

Periodically when the dementia overcame her more deeply, Lillian would cry out for her own mother and be distressed that her Mother wasn't visiting her. Like many in her condition, she'd retreat into her childhood memories and think I was her sister or her favorite niece, Harriet. Mom's early life had been riddled with abandonment and I wondered if she were also reliving her father's dying when she was only seven or the loneliness she'd felt when her siblings left home, leaving her alone with a now busy, hardworking widowed Mom.

This pattern of early "abandonments" had made it difficult for Mom to trust people or develop much self-confidence. But, by the time she'd gotten used to being POParented, Lillian had come to understand that she'd never again be abandoned: I would be with her to the very end! Even without her husband, siblings, or her own mother, I felt she knew that I would be there for her through the remaining years. I so hoped she was able to internalize my love and devotion and finally rest more peacefully.

During her last few years, most of Mom's hospital stays were three to five days long, though occasionally they'd last longer. It felt like a revolving door of admissions and discharges. I wondered how much more her poor body could stand of the routine of coughs, drugs, and hospitals. I appreciated my role as her caring POParent was somewhat limited since, once that plastic bracelet was attached to Lillian's wrist, the hospital ran the show. Nonetheless, I'd learned—as we all eventually find out—that the presence of a family member at an aging person's hospital bedside helps nurses and aides, even doctors, come more quickly and attend more responsively to our loved ones.

So, I would show up, ask my questions, intervene if I could, but, mostly, I was there for her, to hold her hand. Very recently I was listening to Judy Collins sing "In the Twilight," about her own mother's battle with Alzheimer's.[3] It brought streams of tears running down my face, reminding me of those moments when, waking to see me sitting on her hospital bed, my beautiful mom's whole face would light up. "How did you know where to find me?" she'd ask over and again.

Disoriented in a new setting and confused until she saw me, I watched Lillian grow in her gratitude and her happiness in those last years. Now something as everyday as finding herself being attended by the daughter who loved her could bring my mother joy. Since my being there for her seemed to make Mom happy, I wished—fruitlessly—that just showing up was all it would take to keep her healthy, too.

During one of the apparent lulls in hospitalizations, I felt it would be okay to make a short, much-needed trip out of town for business. No sooner had my plane landed in New York than I got a call from her SNF. Mom was moved back to the hospital. I spoke with her physician who reassured me. This pneumonia looked like Mom's other ones, he said, and didn't appear to be life threatening. But I was reminded that these bouts were never easy for Lillian who was just about to turn ninety-five. Based on the doctor's report, I determined to stay the few more days until my planned return.

The afternoon of my return, just as I was about to head over to the hospital, I got a call that Mom's situation had changed dramatically for the worse. I was told that it looked as if she wouldn't make it through the night.

Sighing heavily, I gathered my dearest, and he and I headed north to the hospital in the rush-hour traffic. I remember the crawl of the cars on the 405 Freeway. The string of brake lights stretching ahead seemed interminable. I wondered if we'd arrive there soon enough.

I tried employing my time-tested tools to get calmer—breathing deeply, keeping focused, staying in the present and not anticipating what hadn't yet happened. It was tough going for me during that timeless drive to say goodbye to my mother.

"Tough" was also a good word to describe much of my experience of POParenting Lillian. She'd never been as easy as Jack for me, not since I was a kid. And from the beginning, she had resisted me in everything POP. She hadn't initially wanted to be POParented, to come to California, or to "submit to my will," as she'd put it at the time.

When she finally did come out West and found I didn't run her life, Mom soon warmed to POP, adapting happily to my caring for her. By the time Mom moved to her SNF and away from Dad in the ALF, his health was waning and he had begun withdrawing from her emotionally. He was always fatigued and seemed relieved to transfer to me most of the physical and emotional caregiving he'd been giving my mother for their many decades. I did fill in for him in caring for her, and, after his demise, I was "it."

Then, for these last two and a half years, Lillian and I had "toughed" it out together. I had a particularly difficult time when Mom didn't remember me or was otherwise behaving oddly. Sometimes, when it was hard to face what she and her life had become, I'd even ask my friend Sue to accompany me there. Everybody doing POParenting should be lucky enough to have a great support person like Sue live geographically so well suited to their aging parents. Now, in Mom's apparently final hours, it was Sue I phoned, requesting that she join in, one last time as we waited for the end that was becoming more and more certain.[4]

Despite the many ways Mom had tried to find happiness, which had included good psychotherapy, medication, taking courses, immersing herself in her husband's and then her daughter's life, or volunteering her time in service to causes she believed in, little seemed to result in her true serenity. Still, over our POP time, I'd seen her grow to be genuinely appreciative and more confident with the knowledge that I was POParenting her.

Funny the thoughts that come to us at a moment like this. Driving to the hospital I considered: now that Mom's life was ebbing, there'd be no more time for her to become any happier. By the time we arrived at the hospital and located her in the ER, Mom was already comatose. She lay quietly throughout that evening, never rousing again.

Her delicate, remarkably unlined skin was now pasty white, and she was cold to my touch. Electronic buzzers continually interrupted anything resembling reverential reverie. Unlike Dad's peaceful room at home, the hospital setting offered coldness and confusion. Her environment was agitated with bustling medical staff in their colorful uniforms and the noises of machinery that seemed to be doing little good for her.

People prodded her, poked her, took readings, and made copious notes. More people walked into and out of her area. They looked at Mom, adjusted her machines, said nothing, and left. I asked all the questions I could think of, but still I knew little of what to expect or when.

After a few hours, which felt like weeks, two orderlies wheeled Mom into a more private room. There, for the first time all night, we were allowed to stand close to her, hold her hand, and mop her brow. But the setting was unbearably cold and antiseptic.

Lillian was quietly but definitely failing. I lacked the skill to read the stages her body was going through, but all the trained medical eyes were darting back and forth between Mom's face and the monitoring machines. She looked unbearably fragile and small and particularly unprotected despite all the people and monitors. I wondered how long she could hold on.

I tried to imagine what my mother was thinking or if she were able to compose thoughts at all at this point. I wondered if she were still working on whatever unresolved issues she had right before her earthly end, as I'd been advised by Rick's girlfriend that Dad did. At one point a nurse came by to give Mom her late nightly medication and I sent her away. "Please leave her in peace," I said quietly.

Lillian Wolf would no longer need her medications, not tonight and not any other night ever again. "Are you willing to sign for that?" the nurse wanted to know. Of course, the hospital needed to protect itself legally. I understood. "I will authorize you to stop medicating my mother. She has so little time left; please just let her be in peace, please," I now said with more force. The last hour or two of Mom's life passed uneventfully. It felt unnatural to demonstrate much emotion in that sterile hospital setting. Perhaps that was a good thing—making the next moments less filled with public grieving?

I caressed her hands and her face. I hoped she could still hear the sweet words of serenity and love that I whispered in her ears. Knowing it was our last time, I sat on the crisp white bed with the woman who'd birthed and raised me, sacrificed for me, and loved me every day of my life. She'd been with me at my opening breath and here I was with her at her closing one. And then I "willed" Mom to let go of her body and release herself into the peace. I wondered again: could she hear me? Did she have thoughts or feelings at that last moment? Was she finally at peace? I would never know.

Then the machines Mom was attached to commanded our attention with little noises and blinking lights, and we were made aware that she'd stopped breathing. I observed not only that Lillian's body lost its vitality but also that her spirit appeared to have simultaneously disappeared. As with Dad's passing, it was clear she was there no more. Her transition was otherwise a remarkably quiet event and, much like Dad's, hardly visible to the inexperienced eye.

Back in the car, as we drove home on the now empty freeway, I felt as if time had stopped. Almost immediately my thoughts turned to me: the POP role I'd signed up for ten years ago had come to an end. I'd just become an orphan! My second parent's departing had left me without anyone to POParent. No matter how challenging that had been on occasion, I would miss having a parent around to be proud of me or smile up at me like I'd just invented ice cream. And, without Mom, there was no older generation left to buffer the ever-narrowing distance between me and my Maker.

There was an unexpected moment of amazing relief, even exhilaration. My job was done! It almost felt like the day I'd graduated from college or graduate school, having completed a long-sought-after goal. In its way, POP was a project I'd undertaken that had required years of loving, focused attention and hard work. Now that it was done, I allowed myself to feel good about having been consistent, trustworthy, and resourceful.

I'd also begun to recognize that doing POP had allowed me to give Jack and Lillian an unexpected gift of great value: they had developed renewed pride in themselves! Part of the way my parents interpreted POP and my way of POParenting them was that *they* must have done a really good job instilling family values in me. Hence, *they* felt satisfaction in having parented me well. Because the very thing parents cherish the most is being able to be proud of their offspring, my unplanned-for gift, when their "pride and joy" lovingly POParented them, was they got to feel good about themselves.

It wasn't long before I realized however, that, even after my parents were done living, my POP job was still not totally over. Part of what was left was dealing with a lot of paperwork, legal matters, funeral arrangements, and more. There was closing their bank account(s); informing Social Security, IRS, Medicare, and ASCAP; terminating the agreement with the SNF; and then calling the Neptune Society to make arrangements, and much more.

Another part of my remaining POP tasks involved their "stuff." I still had many items of clothing, memorabilia, furniture, and business records to sort out, give away, or keep. When the dust settled on all their belongings, legal formalities, and my immediate emotions, what was left to plow through was my grieving and adjusting to a new life, without parents to parent and, eventually, after some time, discovering the next trajectory for my own life. During the ten years of POP, my parents weren't the only ones to have aged. I, too, had grown—older and hopefully wiser, truly enriched from what my parents and I had shared. I was certainly not the same woman I'd been before POP. Now I'd have the time to apply what I'd learned and become a better "parent" to my loved ones, my community, and myself! Maybe I'd write a book. . . .

YOUR STORY

If you've chosen to do POP, it's likely you'll have to face the death of at least one aging loved one you've been POParenting. It is a deeply profound experience to attend the passage of your own parents from this planet, regardless of what cultural background you come from, whether you're single or married, are an only child or someone with siblings. As a result, this is the time you'll need to take special care with your parents and yourself.

If you can be present when your parents make their passage, it's likely you will wish to do so. No matter how sad or difficult your parent's death might be for you, it can still be a blessing to attend the remarkable final life passage of someone who con-ceived, birthed, and nurtured you. If you have sufficient time and resources to gather family members and other loved ones from the four corners, you may want to organize a lovely tribute for their concluding days. Of course, such a plan requires you to know when and where their deaths will occur and that's not ordinarily possible.

If you've given yourself the chance to be their POParents, to comfort their final emotional and physical concerns, then you will also get to observe the profound moment of separation between life and death. It is a remarkable experience. What you have always considered your parents' essence seems to also depart, leaving behind cold empty vessels.

Having talked with people who were unable to be present at the end, I have heard stories of their unnecessarily, albeit painfully, carrying around guilt and regret for years. Although it may be optimal to be there when your parents are taking their last breaths, nonetheless, sometimes that will be impossible. Your parent may leave his or her body in an ambulance on the freeway or at some other time and place when you simply can't be there. If that is you, after you have processed your grief, try not to hold on to any painful feelings.

You can only be where you are and you can only give what you've got. Even though you want to act perfectly—just as when you're parenting your children—you're still human. Sometimes you will disappoint yourself and others. But you do the best you can, and carrying around baggage about it doesn't help anyone.

What you should *not* do is to hold on to regrets or resentments about your POPcycle, especially since it's likely you have greatly enriched your parents' lives by doing POP. Regrets and resentments are two of the most effective ways to program yourself for unhappiness. At this uniquely vulnerable time, it's best to avoid these and all other self-destructive sentiments.

Instead, as your final tribute to your parents, you'll want to handle the details around their deaths with grace and thoughtfulness. Maybe you can discover some little things you can do that will actually make a huge difference to your parents' final days and also to the memories that others will hold of your parents as well. For example, I've seen POParents gather the people who'd want a last visit with their parents while they're still alive, for a kind of going-away celebration. Other aging parents might want to reconcile with an estranged sibling. You can arrange, as I did, to reunite couples who've been separated (due to differing levels of aging, an

illness, or some other reason) for their last moments of togetherness.

Arranging these types of get-togethers can be very meaningful,
both for your parents and for those who've loved them. Saying
their proper farewells will allow some of your parents to go more
peaceably. Your thoughtfulness in these areas can tap into the
remarkable healing power in forgiveness and be transformative
experiences for all concerned.

You might customize other fitting tributes for your parents.
This might take the form of honors, awards, plaques, or other
memorial statements that reflect your parents' contributions to the
communities in which they lived, loved, and served. Since your
parents gave of themselves to their work, clubs, families, charitable organizations, religious organizations, and the like, you may
wish to have them take note of your parents' lives (or deaths) and
honor them in some special way. You may particularly want the
younger generations who never knew your parents that well to
learn more about their ancestors, your parents.

When it was "Jack's turn" to be honored, I waited until we held
our memorial celebration event to give him an on-air tribute. I
called the Los Angeles radio station that plays "The Music of Your
Life" format and requested they say some "nice words" about his
songs and play some of the songs my parents used to dance to and
others that Dad had written. I still remember it. In retrospect, I
wish I'd done that when he was still alive.

If you and your siblings are still engaging in contests at this
point in your POPcycle, this could be your time to get better
aligned by putting the unpleasant past behind all of you. Some
POParents find it healing and unifying to sit with family and share
stories as they compose an obituary or other appropriate means of
honoring their parents. Other siblings, far-flung from each other,
may collectively create such eulogies on email. You can use this
meaningful time in life and these types of experiences to heal your
old wounds.

If you would feel good about it, you can also post the POP
music you've come to love and other symbolic statements that

express the ways your parents distinguished themselves to the website's blog at http://www.ParentingOurParents.org.

If it makes sense to you, I encourage you to celebrate your parents while they can still understand and appreciate your accolades and acknowledgments. Honor that they've lived full lives and concentrate on the good feelings that evokes. It is important to remind yourself to have a good time while you're doing POP: just like raising kids, POParenting will be over sooner than you think. And if possible, rejoice even at its conclusion.

Most of us in the Western world have similar reactions to hearing about death: it's horrible and to be feared and avoided at all costs. Your experience, like mine, may well be to the contrary. Death is often a welcome relief for those who've lived well and then spent a lengthy time in a deteriorating physical body. We POParents aren't always willing or able to hear that. When Jack chose to be put on hospice, I had to face that issue, whether or not I liked it. Doing so helped me to understand what he and so many other seniors were saying to their loving POParents: you don't need to mourn for the conclusion of my long and happy life.

Instead of traditional grieving, you might substitute basking in the recognition of how much you've helped your parents feel and function as well as they did during their sunset days. By choosing to POParent them as you did, you supplied your folks with additional reasons to feel satisfied with their lives and accomplishments, including being good mentors to you. They may even see your POParenting as the crowning achievement of their own parenting.

Rather than focusing on your losses, you might gain more serenity by deciding your parents are finally peaceful. After all, the fullness of a life well lived could leave you enriched. A poet offers us this insight:

> Though nothing can bring back the hour
> Of splendour in the grass,
> Of glory in the flower,
> We will grieve not, rather find

Strength in what remains behind.[5]

You need not limit your celebration of your parents to a single time or method. Perhaps you'll even choose to do things backwards, like eating dessert first. For example, during the earlier stages of your POPcycle, when everyone can actively participate, you could arrange a wonderful POP party to honor your parents, show them your gratitude, and make sure your grandchildren get to know your parents better. After their deaths you can host another event, a memorial or a funeral as fits your beliefs, to show your respects.

17

WHEN POP IS OVER AND WE NEED TO LAUNCH OUR NEW LIVES

MY STORY

The ultimate objective of POP was to get my parents safely across the earthly "finish line" with minimal discomfort and maximum serenity. Much time has now passed, it seems, since my father and then my mother departed. Some days I can still hear their voices and almost see them before me. My life is very different without them here, post-POP. In fact, I was changed forever when I chose to parent my parents. I'm so grateful I did.

When I was POParenting them, although the three of us lived in expectation of it, death was never really discussed. How differently my generation has interacted with our kids and our friends! Maybe we went too far in the other direction, sharing too much about our feelings with our children? We thought we were applying the notions we'd learned in our physics classes, that nothing disappears: matter turns into energy. For many baby boomers and others, when important words or feelings are left unexpressed, they only go "underground" and, if unresolved, return later in unexpected formats and time frames.

But in our parents' generation, much was left unsaid. Dad and I had spoken, of course, about my arranging for hospice but never really of his passing or his view of an afterlife. Sometimes not talking about hard topics such as their dying was simpler for me as well as them, apparently, but this absence of discussion left a void.

Mostly in the book I've used the word "transition," which I prefer to "death" because it's better aligned with my beliefs. I believe that our souls are on a journey without end and continue on after our mortal bodies have turned to dust. From my spiritual perspective, it was as if our little family had been running some long-distance marathon together for my whole life. Our pace slowed during the last phase, the POPcycle, as my parents headed toward the completion of their earthly time. And so, Jack and then Lillian's final breaths were contemporaneous with their souls' successfully crossing the finish line. The next steps of their journeys would be taken alone. I could no longer protect them from whatever they might encounter nor share in the joy and peace I hoped they'd now found.

Like so many POParents, while they were still alive, I'd spent time prematurely grieving for Lillian and Jack. I'd even anticipated how my life might change after they'd moved on. To their credit, and reflecting their wisdom, they'd discouraged my fears about the future, reminding me to stay in the present. "We're not dead yet, Jane," they'd commented one day when I was particularly "pre-nostalgic" and a bit weepy.

In the aftermath of their transitions, of course, I was left with an immediate void in my life. But unlike many who'd given up careers, jobs, and homes to attend to their aging parents, much of my pre-POP life seemed to be still intact. I felt fortunate about that, expecting I could pick up where I'd left off before that Christmas a decade ago changed everything. Surely, I'd now have more time to be with my patients and family, more energy for me.

I told myself it was just as natural to launch our children toward college, marriage, or their first home as it was to send off our aged parents to their hereafters. However, no matter how normal, predictable, or expected this was supposed to be in theory, when it was my parents departing, nothing felt normal or comfortable. It felt more like there was a hole in my heart that might never be filled again. Throughout history, sages have consistently offered one adage about grief: time heals. I clearly would need some time.

Immediately after my parents' transitions, there was another flurry of POP activity. There were things to do. I had legal work, banking, Social Security, and Medicare—POP paperwork galore. I had to go through their possessions in their residences and decide what to keep and what to give away. Although I did these final jobs with care, it was more like I was going through the motions, since my heart just wasn't in it. Without Mom or Dad around, doing these tasks felt very different than when they were here, less relevant or important.

Soon I was POP-free. With no parents to care for, I could continue keeping busy, and a part of me definitely wanted to do that. But since those goodbyes at college I'd been ruminating about the time our family would end, and now that the time had come, I needed to stop doing and spend some time just being with my feelings and myself. I wanted to give myself all the time I needed to salve my wounds.

Even with my grieving, I had a way in which I wanted to conduct myself. I'd seen some people lose themselves in their grieving, and I didn't wish to wander aimlessly and endlessly through sad thoughts. My end goal was to live in the present fully. In order to do that, I knew I couldn't go into denial but would need to feel my emotions as deeply as possible and do so when they were still freshest. And yes, I even allowed myself some self-pity about my loss. Later, when I felt more complete about my losses and, hopefully, appreciated some of my gains from POP, I wanted to allow the feelings to depart or, at least, find a useful place to reside inside me.

After both of my parents' transitions, my immediate and predominant feelings had been fatigue, relief, numbness, and—in spite of knowing they had lived full lives—gnawing grief. A part of me felt abandoned, in spite of knowing that my parents' passing wasn't "about me." Although I was already a mature woman and my folks were very old, that didn't matter in that moment.

My grief seemed to be triggered by just a thought, a smell, very often by the sound of a song. It had no regard for whatever I was otherwise doing at the time, sometimes even interrupting me when I was at work. My reactions seemed to rise and fall in waves, rushing over me unexpectedly, and I told myself, rather dramatically, that my life would never be the same. POP seemed to have become a metaphor for life's only constancy, change. When I would tell myself, as a comforting thought, that nothing alive ever stays the same, my mind wanted to answer: what will remain the same hereafter is that I'll never be anyone's daughter again. In those self-pitying moments I found that anything could generate my feeling sorry for my parentless state.

My beloved would respond to that by calling me "the Orphan." It was his way of offering me a hand up and out from this sorrow and these unwarranted conclusions by means of our shared sense of humor. I didn't need to be called "the Orphan" too many times to get the point. I was neither a sad dejected child stranded without her parents nor a soul bereft without a loving connection to the universe. That just wasn't the real me.

In those moments, my mate understood me better than I did. He understood that, when I was thinking more clearly and not overwhelmed with grieving, I would think it was silly, too, and maybe even damaging to view myself in that way. When I wasn't temporarily blinded with sad feelings, I was better able to feel the love I had from so many people, both related and unrelated to me—dead and alive. His faith in me inspired me to come back to myself: I could never be an orphan, an unloved and abandoned person, not unless I chose to put that label on myself.

When, from time to time, I still felt lonely for Mom and Dad, maybe a bit like an orphan, I was usually able to remind myself fairly quickly by focusing on the extraordinary love that I still had every day in my life. I employed my rational, reframed thinking tool to notice: I was neither a child nor in need of protection. In truth, Lillian hadn't functioned as my mother for many years; it was I who had acted as hers.

When I separated myself from these overly emotional and inaccurate thoughts, I was careful to not disavow my authentic feelings of mourning and loss, since I realized they were necessary and appropriate. I also found anger and disappointment interspersed among my other emotions. These were occasionally confusing. Although I knew from clinical research that such feelings often emerge, I'd asked myself: Anger, what's that about? What am I angry about? Then I would comfort myself with its normality: anyone who'd loved and lost might feel angry, confused, and disturbed.

During this process, I did my best to allow myself to feel it all but to react less, to underreact. When I focused on the loneliness and abandonment, inevitably I became unhappy because I'd go back into feeling sorry for myself. This actually deepened my sense of isolation. And when I remembered to breathe into the moment and bring myself back into the present, I always functioned and felt better. I wanted to be experiencing my life through a healthy balance of owning my emotions but not wallowing in them, so I breathed a lot more.

With the realization that the weight of POP's responsibilities was lifting came an unexpected sense of relief, something akin to freedom. For so many years, it had felt oddly normal to be constantly concerned about my parents' well-being. With their transitions, I'd gotten a reprieve from that worry and releasing it altogether would help me take the first steps in the direction of my "new life."

No longer on call 24/7, 365 days a year for Jack and Lillian, I could now let my phone go unanswered until I felt available to be interrupted. As a mental health professional, I'd always been reachable, but now, knowing I wouldn't be missing a time-critical POP message, I could check later. Right after savoring that exhilaration, I thought I heard Janis Joplin croon: "Freedom's just another word for nothing left to lose."[1] How complicated grief really is!

Since my birth I'd been part of the Wolf triangle, with each of us needed to complete the whole. After Mom's dementia set in and her hip condition required my parents to live separately, I'd experienced the loss of their "coupleness" as weakening our triangle. When I drove Dad to spend time with Mom, the three of us would sit together in her room or go out to the skilled nursing facility's (SNF's) garden. Then I'd momentarily recapture a childhood fantasy—that our family was invincible and timeless—only to come back sharply into the present day.

I had now become the historian of the Wolf family, as well as keeper of all its possessions. I felt inexplicably dislocated. As an only child, I always knew that my parents would one day leave me here "alone," but, I was only now learning what that really meant. From now on, only I would laugh at our inside jokes and understand the familiar references we'd spent our earlier lives together creating.

On some occasions I saw my grief resulting in questioning my POP performance, evaluating the choices I'd made and those I'd declined. Fortunately, my spiritual tradition invited me to think about these things in a more neutral way, rather than to judge or blame myself for things I could no longer change. I also comforted myself with the thought that I'd done my best at POParenting, the best I knew how—given who I was and what I had to work with at the time.

Facing my parents' mortality required me to face my own as well. In turn, thinking about my own death led me to examine my life and contributions. What had my life, up until this time, been all about? What were my core values and was I living by them? When I left the planet, how would I wish to be remembered?

Throughout our POPcycle, I'd periodically wondered: where will I be spending my senior years? Would I inherit my mother's dementia? Would I request to be put on hospice like Jack had done? Might I spend my final days in a facility staring off into space? Or would I be like my Aunt Frieda, who played her last round of golf at eighty-eight, walked off the fairway, and immediately expired? Would I be the healthy senior enjoying life and loved ones and contributing right up to the end, as I hoped?

Seeing it from this vantage point, POP seemed to involve a lot of consideration about my own aging and me. It was almost as if my involvement with POP was a rehearsal for my own old age. When I'd gone to look at senior residential facilities for my folks, I'd often pictured the scene, years ahead, when I'd be the prospective resident. Without even being conscious of it, entering a facility's front door, I'd be asking myself: if it were me, would I want to live here? Years from now, who would scout facilities for me?

With their passing, I saw my parents' absence from the planet and my life in yet another context. It was now my generation who'd become the heads of families. Gone was the "buffer layer" between my Maker and me: we were "next up." I even wondered if my parents were continuing to watch over me now that they'd crossed over to some other plane.

As time wore on, my memories of Lillian and Jack grew a bit dimmer. Even my vision of them as old people was fading, and in my mind's eye, sometimes they were young again. It seemed I was less sad when I remembered them as vibrant. As the days continued, thoughts about Mom and Dad would bring a smile more often than a tear.

I longed to hold on to those smile-making memories and the sweet recollection of things I'd experienced doing POP, and there were many. An offering from the Buddha helped me remember how much control lay in how I thought about my experiences. "Your worst enemy cannot harm you as much as your own thoughts unguarded. But once mastered, no one can help you as much, not even your father or your mother." I practiced this advice, guarding against engaging with disturbing thoughts as I did when I meditated. Instead, I'd practice the technique of evaluating them for their irrationality and letting them go.

As time passed, the challenging feelings became less intense. Gradually, as I began to feel in greater control, I wondered: What would my post-POP healing look like? Even if it occasionally upset me to remember my parents, I didn't want to banish my memories of them. I tried permitting myself to bask in the warmth of my happy remembrances. Recovering from the loss of POP could look differently than I'd expected—more like permitting the memories to come up naturally—and knowing some might trigger pride and joy, while others might bring on my nostalgia. I sought to proactively evoke comforting thoughts, insights, and recollections because those led me to feel lighter emotionally. On occasion I'd aim to recall something specific and positive, like my parents' satisfaction when I graduated from college or the way Mom's face would beam when I'd done some POP kindness for her. As time went on, even childhood memories—like Dad teaching me lyrics to his latest song—could source my smiles.

I came to see my parents' transitions as part of a larger irony in the human condition: we live and die in our solitariness as well as in our connectedness. We come onto the planet apparently alone, hopefully make deep human connections that we'll eventually need to leave, and pass off the planet, apparently alone again. My spiritual perspective refuted the notion that the appearance of aloneness was reality, offering me the view that we are always with God.

It also suggested that there was a major difference between losing my parents because they'd left the planet and they're being "lost" to me. I still retained my memories of Jack and Lillian and their vast influence on my life. Since that was so, I reasoned, I could find my parents whenever I wished. They weren't lost—they'd simply moved on.

Time continued to pass, and my emotions kept coming and going in waves, but for the most part, the more intense ones diminished in size and potency. Then, out of the blue, some powerful memory would wash over me and I'd be overwhelmed with tears and feelings of loss or, sometimes, laughter. In an instant I could be that child again, back with my parents when we'd all been younger together.

One day, an Elton John song about his father came on the car radio. I was suddenly Daddy's little girl all over again. We are dancing. My small arms are reaching up toward his faraway shoulders and my feet are planted on top of his. That vision seemed to stop my heart in its tracks; I pulled off the road to sit and weep.

Even though Mom and Dad are now long gone, I sometimes find myself musing, "Wouldn't Mom love this beautiful museum exhibit? I want to bring her here." Or I think, "I can't wait to tell Dad about that." Randomly, I find myself quoting one of Jack's many witticisms. When I see something that's clearly outrageously priced, I notice Jack's voice ironically saying: "Rich or poor, Jane, it's nice to have money." Other times, I catch a glimpse in the mirror of my resemblance to Lillian and think: I *am* my mother's daughter.

Some days I get the notion to carry around a little piece of Lillian or Jack with me for support, comfort, or good luck. I'll put on a special pin Mom bought me, a piece of clothing that belonged to her or one she knit for me back in the day. Or I'll be driving and decide to play a song of Jack's and sing along with the words he taught me. I recognize these gestures as symbols of my ongoing healing process. They are small sacred steps, refilling the emptier parts that remain in my heart and honoring my parents' memories as I savor the special influence each of them had on me.

I admit to sometimes feeling envious of people who still have living parents. Father's Day and Mother's Day are predictably challenging for me. Even seeing an adult woman strolling arm in arm down the street with her mom occasionally triggers reactions similar to those I had in my more immediate post-POP days.

As my little rescued puppy became increasingly older and frailer, I noticed I'd started associating my dog's last days with my parents' end on the planet. The pet I'd brought over to be with Dad on his last day was himself becoming too weak to reach down to eat food or drink water. I feared that my eighteen-year-old dog's imminent demise could stimulate another wave of grieving. Instead of going to that place, I tried to examine my thoughts with a clearer lens and distinguish my feelings about him from those about my parents. I had to literally say to myself: "This is your dog, Jane, not your Dad or Mom," and I needed to remind myself of that reality more than once.

I also reminded myself how long and wonderful the dog's life had been. This mode of thinking brought me into a different quality of mourning about him, one similar to thinking about how my parents had lived lengthy and robust lives, where I wasn't so much saddened as tearful with appreciation, honoring a life well and fully lived. Afterward, I was better able to hold on to that more rational reframe. Doing so added to my strength, making it easier to appropriately end my dog's suffering. At his end, he too left the planet, serene in my arms.

It took me yet another year after Mom's departure to put together the POP-concluding celebration of my parents' lives that I wanted to hold. I invited those people who were closest to me to my near-oceanfront home and decorated the library with symbols of my parents' accomplishments. I displayed Jack's statewide athletic trophies, some unique objects of art Lillian had designed, and lots of their memorabilia. I enlarged a photo of the three of us to poster size. In it my parents are sitting around their little girl and they are vibrantly, beautifully youthful! The man who bought my father's music publishing made a special CD of his songs for the celebration, so our favorite Jack Wolf songs provided the background music as conversation focused on my days of doing POP. In the foreground Benny Mardones, a singer friend with an amazing voice, crooned Dad's tunes for us. Even though some people there had never met my parents, few eyes remained dry that afternoon.

The final step I'd planned was to release a portion of their ashes into the welcoming waters of the Pacific after my beloved minister friend Sue offered us powerful words of spiritual inspiration. I asked everyone to grab a balloon and a marker, write a special message on it to Jack and Lillian and carry it to the ocean where we'd let the messaged balloons ascend into the heavens.

Meanwhile I'd brought along two beautiful champagne flutes that I'd filled with some ashes from each of their urns for this ceremonial walk. When the processional arrived at the water and the words were said, I emptied the flutes and watched the contents mix together as I invited the sea to have its way with their remains. Like so many POPlans, this last one—to release the balloons overhead—met with some unexpected resistance. One of our invited guests was the Los Angeles police chief; he said that we couldn't send off our balloons with their sweet messages as they posed a hazard to LA Airport's congested airspace. The irony of seeing a part of my final POPlan dissolve in front of my eyes was hardly lost on me.

And after that, POP was over.

It hit home more poignantly than ever that everyone I love comes into and out of my life so quickly. Therefore, the most important POP lesson for me is to live joyously with those we cherish during the time we have with them. That core realization continues to guide me as I help my patients, loved ones, and those whom I coach to live their POPcycle and the remainder of their lives with more joy.

Recently I was sitting with a patient. She is a forty-four-year-old woman who has unexpectedly been called upon to care for her seventy-three-year-old father with advanced Parkinson's. Their history together had been occasionally stormy but she's working with me, in part, to become a more patient POParent. On this day she was furious with her father over some incident she's unlikely to recall for long. I asked her a question and later I realized that it had emerged from my current view of POP. "If you were told your dad had only six months to live, how might knowing that alter your anger today?" She stopped and thought about it. "What I'm so mad about probably wouldn't matter at all to me, then."

She paused, and I saw a light of recognition appear from deep within this woman's eyes. Then we both heard her enlightened response. "What would really matter would be to best love the man my dad is today and forgive the man he is no longer. I suppose I can let go of the anger I'm feeling today too, since it's not rage but love I wish to grow between him and me." I could see that, for her as for me, POParenting often resulted in healing.

Thinking about my aging and my own future, I found myself posing Oprah's great question. "What is it, Jane, that you know for sure?" My answer is: I know that I don't need to plague myself with scary thoughts of being homeless, impoverished, unloved, or disabled in my senior years. These are not what I foresee for myself or intend to ever let happen.

I can never know what's ahead. But I needn't add worrying to my not knowing; I can just admit that tsunamis, companies not paying pensions, Ponzi schemes, and unknowable unknowns can change everything. I also don't know for sure that I would ever wish the younger generation to bear the awesome responsibilities my parents entrusted to me. But I *do* wonder what lessons and conclusions the people in those younger generations are reaching, having witnessed their parents doing POP.

For myself, it' likely I'll want to find—or maybe create—an intentional community where I'll age alongside my beloved and other like-minded friends who've essentially become our second family. Maybe I'll want to age in place in my own home. Maybe something completely unexpected will occur. Once I decide which direction to go in, I'll need to consider what steps I should be taking financially, legally, emotionally, and spiritually in order to ensure that my choices will eventually occur.

As I look back over my life thus far, I find that little has helped me to grow up faster than parenting. Learning how to "be the grown-up," first in my twenties with my stepchildren and later, in midlife, with my own parents, brought out the most adult and, at other times, the most childish parts in me. Both parenting opportunities advanced me giant steps toward becoming more nurturing, compassionate, and patient and, I can only hope, my clients, my loved ones, and I will be ongoing beneficiaries of that. I expect that you're noticing, too, that your compassion and other qualities that you need the most expanding as you move through your POP-cycle.

What I've aimed to do in this book is to empower you to create your own best version of a good POPcycle by sharing my own, however flawed it was and however different from yours it may appear to be. I stated in the beginning that such private revelations have challenged me, but it was well worth it if my story helps you develop more competence and confidence in constructing your best version of POP.

As I noted earlier, you're likely to discover how alike we all are when we're doing POP. Just stand in line at your grocery store with a package of adult diapers and see how quickly another POP-arent will engage you in conversation about your POP story and theirs. It's likely you're making many different POP choices for your parents than I made for mine or than the person at the market has made. And that's how it should be. This book is not about following the same options I chose for Lillian and Jack. No path is the right one for all.

We in this POP generation are each part of a bigger community. Our numerous opportunities for loving, healing, and giving span across nations, cultures, and families. You and I are among tens of millions of POParents who now spend time with our parents, seek forgiveness, get do-overs, invoke gratitude, savor today's goodness, and reverse the roles from our childhood with our parents.

I began to notice how universal POP was when total strangers, people whose names I never learned, shot me what I came to call the "POP look." I'd be doing something small for Mom and Dad, like patiently getting them in or out of my car or adjusting a scarf for one of them against the cold, when I'd be flashed this warm sign of recognition, even faint approval. I got the POP look more often as Jack and Lillian "advanced" from walking upright to needing canes, then walkers to lean on and, finally, to being pushed in their wheelchairs as they'd pushed me in my stroller.

Most often this POP look came to me from my peers, middle-aged men and women, but not always. They seemed to be offering me a silent blessing in their POP look. It was a powerful connection because it meant that another person, perhaps a POParent, got what POP was and what we were doing here together. The POP look startled me with its unexpected depth of camaraderie, and each time, I experienced an emotional warmth, a connection, that I'll never forget. Now that my POP days are over, I miss receiving it, but I still give the POP look to other POParents repeatedly every day! In its way, it was the universality I felt, getting the POP look, that helped me birth the idea of the global POP community you and I are currently constructing together here, online at the POP website and wherever else we are traveling.

To answer Oprah's fascinating question with regard to my POP journey, I know this for sure: I received far more by doing POP than I ever gave. Together my parents and I shared the opening and closing of the Circle of Life, and somehow we created a beautiful love story.

It is because I parented Lillian and Jack that I also know this for sure: I don't want any of you to go through more of your POPcycle without the community you need to help you do it well. Read on in the book's epilogue to see where we go from here and what's next. What we need to accomplish this demanding work in a satisfying and loving way is here. Parenting Our Parents is growing exponentially, one family at a time, with every family and every POP story welcome!

THEIR STORY—DAD

Jane honey, I want you to have the benefit of everything I've come to understand during my lifetime. Gosh, can you believe it? I've had ninety-two years of so much richness and so much living?

First, Jane, you've got to know how very proud I am of you! Your Mom and I both have been for years. I told you that many times and I hope I've told you often enough. I'll happily tell you again now: you were a wonderfully devoted daughter. When we got old and needed you to help us, you took consistently good care of your Mom and me. And, if anyone knows, I do—we weren't always easy.

Second, I'm okay with everything. Specifically, I'm just fine with your writing a book that we're all in that can help other families do even better, after they read what our family went through. Privacy can be greatly overrated, especially after you've gotten old. I'm better than "just fine" with your writing this book. I highly approve of the project because so many people desperately need help parenting their parents.

People need your help. You've had so many relevant life experiences, studied law and psychology, physiology, and philosophy and integrated it all to become who you are now: a source of comfort and "normality" for people parenting their parents! So, anything you deem relevant to include in the book about us, that's all right by me. After all, we writers have got to share what we've learned. And, by the way, my dear daughter, congratulations on becoming a writer—your grandmother, Uncle George, and I will all want to take credit for your choice, I'm sure.

Third, you'll remember my always telling you that living well came down to a few basics. Turns out that your old Dad was smarter than either of us knew, or at least about that, honey. Human life is simple. Ultimately, it's about love, joy, and contribution. As I have been closer to leaving my body, I've developed an appreciation for how hard it is to be in a human body while it ages. Although our senses are gifts to enjoy the human experience, once they start to go, it becomes challenging to live as fully. It became hard not to focus on the changes I was seeing in Lillian and me too. Frankly, the planet on the whole seems very different to me now than when I was younger. Damned shame, so many people I've loved are already gone, and then there's your Mom. She's almost worse than dead—looking and sounding like herself but not really my Lillian any more.

Aging felt like a long string of losses. For the first time in my life, an overwhelming sadness descended over me. My God, I even tried to end my life three times. And Jane, I am *so* sorry for those attempts and how my forgetting the joy of living may have hurt you. Thank you for saving me from myself! From my current vantage point, I see again that life is grand but not unless I actually enjoy it. So, my darling daughter, it's time for us both to become peaceful, give up any struggles we may carry, and enjoy what shows up.

I expect there may be pain during this upcoming passage. Hopefully I won't feel it except maybe the sorrow of watching your face as my body leaves Earth and you for the last time. But do not grieve because that will be my last moment ever of human sadness. Thereafter, I'll be free of all the body's pains and aging. In my next life, I will be new again.

I want you to always feel the love I have for you, no matter my form or yours. Those of us for whom you sacrificed when doing POP thank you for our sunset years! We will love you forever and we hope that you healed yourself as much as you helped us to heal. As far as I know, you're right in thinking that your mother and I will never be "lost" to you nor you to us, not even after we leave this planet. But, after all, you did inherit my intelligence. Soon you'll also be inheriting my membership in ASCAP, the songwriters' and publishers' association, and I love that you'll receive my ongoing love reminders in the form of royalties from the music I wrote.

Speaking of music, I hear it's gloriously musical on the other side, Jane! Maybe there's an ongoing vibration that's harmonic and magnificently peaceful. . . . Life after the life I gave you may be even better than life on earth. Death seems to be its own beginning rather than a final ending. Not only that but, where I'm going, I won't need those damned thickeners and can finally get a decent cup of Joe. I'm thinking it will be sweet there, hopefully with other spirits I've loved, throughout eternity.

And Jane, one last time, my dear daughter, thank you for being in my life! I love you!

YOUR STORY

With the passing of a parent, each of you will be required to make changes, one last time. Every POParent grieves in a unique and special way. There is no right or wrong to it. Bereavement experts report there are many different types of losses, everything from the loss of faith to the loss of limb. You can lose your parents, children, pets, health, friends, and your money. You can lose your way, your sense of values, misplace your things, and even lose the companionship of other people. People process their losses and specifically their good-byes in a wide variety of ways. Some deny, some regret, some pine away. The loss of an aging parent may be predictable but does that mean it isn't painful or that it hurts you any less than if your parents had died when you were younger?

After your POPcycle is completed and while you're contemplating what you've lost, you can also discover who you've become, as a result of participating in this extraordinary and transforming experience with your aging loved ones. Soon you may be asking yourself: Since I've fulfilled my POP mission, what do I want next? But that time is not quite upon you yet. First you must take a bunch of deep and cleansing breaths, discover where you're at now, rest up for a while, and regroup. All of this may take some time. If you give yourselves sufficient therapeutic time now, it's likely you'll complete your healing more thoroughly and you won't need to deal with it again later.

The end of a POPcycle represents many different things, depending, of course, on how you choose to look at it. If you're like most people, you'll soon be focusing a lot of attention on how much you've lost. Your friends may see it as their new job to listen empathically as you recount what you no longer have. For those of you who substantially rearranged your lives to accommodate POP-arenting—moved away from your home to stay with them, given up your full-time job—your losses may now include the POP life you've created, its accompanying lifestyle, and maybe even your recent self-identification.

Not only have you been deprived of your parents' companionship—and the various consequences that may have—but you've also been left without your recent central responsibility and, perhaps, your reason for getting up in the morning for some years. Certainly, you've lost the satisfaction gained from performing helpful POP tasks, watching your folks enjoy your giving to them, and a myriad of other good things that joined your life with theirs. Some of you may find yourself grieving, as I did, for the loss of your original nuclear family and the absence of your parents' "coupleness." You may be feeling emotional losses reflecting your sense of abandonment at being left behind as the sole family historian or with siblings you never liked that much.

Can you interpret your losses in an empowering way, rather than being overwhelmingly sad over loved ones no longer here? Yes, you can try to place your attention on being grateful for all your positive POP times and rewarding opportunities. Think about all you've gained from the last years or months you had with them. Concentrate on your having been there for them at the end or resolving your differences and finally knowing they were proud of you. You could even be thankful that you've lost some things you're happy to be rid of, like dealing with their Social Security and Medicare problems, accommodating your schedules to your parents' needs, or worrying about them.

Certainly, the parents who saw you attend to them so lovingly wouldn't want you to suffer for long after they'd gone. Instead of struggle and strife, you can adopt a more uplifting point of view. For example, remind yourself that since completing POP, you have more space and time opened up to explore new things, that all endings can be seen as beginnings for other things. By making that type of mental fix, it will become easier to gain your desired closure on POP.

When you stopped taking care of your children, you found more time for your hobbies or to return to school. Similarly, when you complete your POParenting, you'll have more resources to put into expanding your world in other ways. Perhaps what will unfold ahead will turn out to be your best time yet, the occasion to take up a long-awaited pursuit worthy of your now more available time and energy. Maybe you'll want to become a POP Family Coach and help guide other families from what you've learned.

So how do you move on and let go? What does it mean to "move on?" Let go . . . of what? Since you're not letting go of loving your parents nor moving on from your tender memories of POParenting, how can you let go of your sadness, regrets, resentments, losses, and angers? How do you move on to your next project or even discover what it is? You've been developing useful tools throughout your work with this book. It's time to apply them so you can better manage your feelings of loss and vulnerability and become more resilient and creative again.

Those tools have included: reframing your POP experience to extract the valuable lessons for yourself; forgiving your siblings, your parents, yourself, and whomever else for the "small things" you've done or omitted to do (and that is, most things); practicing the habit of gratitude; remembering there are always things about POP for which you can find some appreciation; savoring your good memories of times long ago and more recently. Working these practices is the road to helping yourself feel more enlivened and energized not only in your POP life but now in your post-POP days as well.

Another secret tool is this: *Learn to make friends with change!* Put differently: by accepting the "now" that you have, you can—and will—complete your grieving sooner and more completely than if you persist in fighting what's so!

By engaging with these tools that utilize your intelligence, you can "reorganize" some reactions into more useful perspectives. You have been expecting your parents' inevitable departures, even if you haven't admitted it, felt okay about it, or known the exact day or cause in advance. You were realistic enough to acknowledge that the time would come when your aged parents would surrender to fatigue, a chronic illness, or some bug making its way around their SNF.

Sooner or later, everyone you love will disappear from the planet, as will you and I. Since longevity is certainly a goal for many, the longer you live, the more losses you will predictably need to face. You have a lot more choice now, because of these tools you've learned from POP, to either suffer through your losses or get through to the other side of grief, with grace and gratitude.

By practicing your POP techniques, hopefully you can avoid repeated "wreckage" when you encounter predictable and inevitable losses. By doing so, you can preserve some of your energy and be less susceptible, emotionally and physically, when such losses occur. You can program yourself to appreciate that, although nature didn't give humans a body that would last forever, you needn't be overly dramatic about it.

Just because mortality is a fact, that doesn't require you to fear the imminent deaths of everyone you love on a daily basis. Nor do you need to evoke the kind of apprehension I did, when your parents leave you "alone" after visiting you at college. How much better to choose fully enjoying the experiences afforded by your friends and relatives when you're all still alive and have each other to enjoy. What a way to live that would be!

Many of you have noticed some very favorable changes in your relationships with your parents since you started doing POP. You may have observed a mellowing in long-held withdrawn emotions or felt a sense of relief and gratitude from your parents that feels boundless. Others may have been disappointed that POP didn't do all you wanted to minimize your differences with your parents and/or your siblings. But your life with them is not over just because POParenting is done.

If you never developed the relationship you wanted with one or both of your parents, their deaths may have made that seem impossible to rectify. But just because you never created the perfect parent-child relationship or didn't achieve all you wanted from doing POP, that doesn't mean you're without options. I've worked with people to heal their relationships with alienated, neglectful, and even abusive parents after the parents were no longer alive. Award-winning novelist Tom Robbins put a different slant on it when he suggested: "It's never too late to have a happy childhood!"[2] Even after your parents have gone, you can forgive them and see how that changes you.

What's it like for those left behind after someone you've parented leaves home? If you ask that question to parents who've recently launched their youngster off to college, the armed forces, marriage, or even to an apartment down the street, you're likely to get one consistent answer: life is very different! Much the same can be said here. Each POParent is likely to feel their parents' absence differently depending on a whole variety of factors, such as: how much you disrupted your former life for POP, whether your post-POP life is fulfilling, and what expectations of POP were never met.

After POP is through, your life *will* be different. Each POParent is likely to feel their parents' absences differently depending on a whole variety of factors, such as: how much you disrupted your former life for POP, whether your post-POP life is fulfilling, and what expectations of POP were never met. If you moved your parents in with you, you may have needed to reorganize your home, built some space for them, or even revamped your life altogether. It's hard to know anyone who's been employed during POP whose work life hasn't been affected by that.

In order to do POP, many of you had to postpone doing things in your careers and jobs that might have influenced your pay, advancement, early retirement, or other benefits. You may or may not be able to jump back into those endeavors or the other plans you'd hoped for and put off—like traveling or going back to school. To pick them back up, you'll need to be able to afford to develop those interests as well as have the stamina to do them now.

Sadly, some of you have carried around unconscious fears of abandonment and neglect from your earliest moments. Others actually were left behind, abused or uncared for during childhood. Some adults retain residual effects of early childhood fears and trauma for their whole lives, creating a mental template where loss seems ever present and even a small loss feels like a major rejection. Graduations, weddings, or other occasions marking the passage of time, which are joyous for many, can be sad for them. Funerals may be unbearable for people with seriously unresolved issues of abandonment.

Even for those of you without such challenging histories, recent losses can trigger the suffering of your earliest and usually most painful losses, whether remembered by you or not. Part of the reason you may cry when you see others experiencing loss is you're reliving similar feelings, even if they're below the level of consciousness. During your most vulnerable times, as when you're grieving, it's easy to pull up the string that binds painful losses together.

Since any hurtful loss can potentially tug on your string, unrelated events in your life seem to look alike and a small loss can feel like an old, deep one. You'll want to be on the alert to these new waves of old grief, since they may feel inexplicably strong. When you've undergone a recent loss, make sure you separate it out from your former losses. For example, it's easy to reach false generalizations that are destructive to you and are usually unwarranted, such as "it's hopeless. I'll always be alone. People have been leaving me since I was born" or "I'd be better off never loving again because (wo)men always abandon me sooner or later."

Discipline your thinking! Train your brain to be your friend! You have been taught many useful tools to help. Now it's your time to apply the tools you've learned and fight the seemingly magnetic pull to feel sorry for yourself. For example, when my dog lay in my arms dying, it was very hugely sad for me, of course. Momentarily, I evoked the memory of being with each of my parents during their transitions, but I was much better off when I could detach the "string" of losses, separate the animal from my parents, and then focus on my gratitude for all the years we'd had together. I was much calmer when I stopped concentrating on the loss and instead savored the memory of his rascal-like behavior and how many times I'd had to rein in his playful ways.

You will want to experience and express the grief you're feeling in the way that's best for you. Some people talk with their intimates; some write in journals; others work out at the gym. It's of little value to compare your way of mourning to others. Disavowing your own pain because someone may have seen greater pain honors no one. You may have lost only a parent and someone else their whole family or a whole village in an earthquake, but one person's sadness can't really be compared to anyone else's.

There are also no time limits on how long it may take you to recover from the demise of someone you've POParented. You can speed up the time you spend living in the sadness however, by working with the tools, insights, and other people who've been where you are in the POPcycle. Your family or others may want you to recover more quickly than feels right to you. They may not know how to cheer you up and are likely to have good motives for wanting you to feel better. They may even acknowledge that, since POP is over, they'd like you to be more present with them. But they may not be the most objective people to evaluate your course of healing.

Sometimes the people who ordinarily support you aren't able to help you much at this time. If your nearest and dearest are concerned you're not snapping back quickly enough, take their remarks seriously and respectfully. They may be correct that you're wallowing in your grief or have become somewhat dysfunctional. Just in case they're right, heed their concern and get yourself checked out by professionals. A therapist, pastoral counselor, POP Family Coach, or even a short-term grief group may help you better assess how well you're resolving your emotions and how to move through the unwanted feelings more quickly.

As you're becoming less overwhelmed with sad feelings and more proficient at managing your loss, try experimenting with bringing out your good memories in a somewhat controlled manner. Interrupt the automatic lonely feeling you get every time you pass the coffee shop you used to take your Dad after his doctor's appointments by trying something different. See if you can recall some happy times with your aging loved ones. Instead of feeling melancholic or pining for the good old days, reach into your bank of positive memories and find one with more enjoyable feelings for you than sadness.

Take a breath and see if you can smile as you fondly recall some sweet moments. Warm yourself with your recollections of how your dad loved his vanilla lattes, blowing on the foam so he wouldn't burn himself and getting it on his nose. As you get more distance from the intensity of your loss, you can be more proactive in encouraging your pleasurable POP memories to become a bigger and better part of your everyday life.

It may help you to complete POP by creating a ceremony to recognize your parents' passing or perhaps the beginning of the end to your mourning. You might like to create the type of small event I did or take private time to think, look at photos, read poetry, or whatever seems appropriate. Use these events to guide yourself into the present, where you can live in the now of your post-POP era.

Remember this: the people you POParented, your parents, would never want you to live indefinitely with your grief. You can tell you're beginning to move on when your sadness lifts, you spend less time every day thinking about your parents and your losses and/or you actually feel more like yourself. Another sign may be that you're looking around, seeking to reinvest yourself again—wondering whether or not, where and how you'll proffer your unique talents in your world. You won't have to look too far to locate people and places where you can continue the circle of giving and receiving you engaged in during POP. Creating your unique loving post-POP gift can transform yourself and your world.

I know you can also make a meaningful contribution by going to http://www.ParentingOurParents.org. There you can join the community of other POParents and senior parents, share your challenges, post about how doing POP has resulted in lessons or information you'd like to teach others and continue to learn and teach more about living happily.

EPILOGUE

Where Do We All Go from Here?

Hopefully this book has been of ongoing assistance, giving you an understanding about how to best structure your POPcycle, whom to include on your POP team, how you want to be as a POParent, and how to know when you need more help. In the future, this book can continue to serve as a reliable place to turn for information and support. Keep it handy on your bookshelf or store it on your tablet to keep informed about the next stage of POParenting you're facing and to calm yourself as you meet your family's next set of challenges. Tell a friend who's struggling!

This book will also do much to help you discover wise responses to those questions and hopefully many more. As you read, you may be thinking about your own "plan of action" regarding POP. It may be that you want to create a POParenting Group at your church, school, or synagogue—a place to learn from others how each of you navigates the treacherous POP waters more peaceably. You may work to have your state update the law and begin court-ordered POP classes to teach better skills as well as to avoid elder abuse. You might be seeking a public program allowing some respite hours to refresh yourself.

As we look around, it seems that however desperately Americans may wish for a comprehensive governmental protective net for seniors, it does not now exist. Nor does it appear that our political leadership is creating new and better solutions to the many POP challenges you and I have been bearing alone all these years. So, if we aren't going to be able to rely on governmental programs, training, and support, where will the help we need come from? How will you and I manage our stressful POP demands at 3 a.m. or even 3 p.m., whenever our parents' situations demand our help?

One thing is for sure. You will *not* be able to do it all alone! Therefore, if help isn't going to come from governmental coffers, and your siblings aren't going to be any less busy or easy to deal with than they have been so far, where will the additional assistance you know you will need to do POParenting well come from? Your help comes from the millions of other Americans who are also doing POP. After all, who else is wide awake worrying at 3 a.m. about Dad's diabetes and his threatened home foreclosure? Who else can you contact who has dealt with the issues you are now facing? The answer is simple: other POParents. How do you find them?

With the publication of this book and the growth of the community at our website (http://www.ParentingOurParents.org), I officially declare: *The nationwide POP community has begun!*

This website is the twenty-first-century equivalent of a huge home for our POP community. Go there to find what you need and to contribute what you already know. You'll have access to everything POP—geriatric links, reviews of services provided to POParents, videos about POP, and a blog with varying points of view. The POP website offers the advantages of social networking but is beyond and different from that. Hopefully being part of this community means that by doing POP we're all part of a bigger whole and you'll never be as alone, scared, uninformed, or isolated again! After all, you're doing POP and are on a mission of love!

When you're lonely and so fried from POP responsibilities that you think you can't make one more decision, I recommend the best thing to do right then and there, 24/7 is: go to the Parenting Our Parents website, the portal for all things POP. A quick sign-up there and you'll become a member of the POP community. You will receive your personal and complimentary VIP invitation to share your POP journey with others.

Once a member of the POP community, you can comment on the blog, meet other POParents who share your particular concerns, and learn about others who might provide you much-needed POP services. Your postings allow you to locate fellow POParents who live near your mom; send a shout-out by means of a great video of your family reunion; get a recommendation from your high school friend in Florida for a caregiver to your favorite uncle, now living alone in Kansas. You can chat there with other POParents, people who get what you're feeling and doing, and can offer some practical advice as well as genuine understanding. Sharing your POP problems and, even better, your POP solutions with people who understand you and your challenges without a lot of unnecessary explanation will get you more than one good night's sleep.

There are countless POParents all over the globe. At this very moment, you have your very same deepest thoughts, worries, and feelings. You just don't know them yet. And they may well have good answers for you. Even if it's 3 a.m. where you are, someone else on the website can assist. In today's global POP community, there will always be POParents awake and ready to help you.

If your personal mission is bringing joy to your family's POPcycle, you will ultimately require three things to succeed: your focused intention; the right equipment; and a robust interactive POP community to help you update your information, get enough support, and share what you have to offer.

Hopefully this book and its accompanying website will get you well on your way to having everything you'll need. However, you may find you wish more personal, direct support from the author. I do offer POP Family Coaching to a limited number of families to help smooth the bumps in the journey.

We can be in your POPcycle together! You can obtain information at the website on how to obtain POP Family Coaching from me as well as how to work with me to become a Certified POP Family Coach yourself. Learning how to use your POP experience to help other families by becoming a Certified POP Family Coach can be very rewarding and a terrific legacy to your parents. Sharing what you've been through with others while earning a good living doing so might be where you go from here.

Perhaps my single best piece of advice is this: don't try POParenting alone! You need companions on your journey since you simply cannot do POP as well by yourself as you can with the support of other POParents. You'll ultimately need to depend not only on your family but also on your friends, your parents' professionals, and even on POParents you've never met before.

As demanding as your POP journey can be, I have never met anyone who regrets having chosen it. When you've transformed your remarkable set of POP challenges into a journey of love, all your relationships hopefully will be filled with more peacefulness and more joy.

NOTES

PROLOGUE

1. That is, healing work done by reading books, articles, and magazines.

2. Benjamin Spock, revised and updated by Robert Needlman, *Dr. Spock's Baby and Child Care*, eighth edition (New York: Pocket Books, 2004).

3. Originally published in 1984 and consistently on the best-seller list. Heidi Murkoff and Sharon Mazel, *What to Expect When You're Expecting*, fifth edition (New York: Workman, 2016).

5. DOING AND UNDOING PAPERWORK

1. It's most prudent to discuss these matters with estate or other qualified lawyers and financial advisors in your parents' home state as these standards vary and are determined by state law.

6. FACING DOWN THE LIFE-AND-DEATH MISSION OF POP— THEIRS AND YOURS

1. National Alliance for Caregiving, Caregiving in the U.S. 2009, a report conducted in collaboration with AARP and funded by the MetLife Foundation (Bethesda, MD: National Alliance for Caregiving), https://www.caregiving.org/data/Caregiving_in_the_US_2009_full_report.pdf.

2. National Alliance for Caregiving, Caregiving in the U.S. 2009.

3. National Institute of Mental Health, "Suicide Prevention," https://www.nimh.nih.gov/health/topics/suicide-prevention/index.shtml#part_153178.

4. Yang Yang, "Social Inequalities in Happiness in the United States, 1972 to 2004: An Age-Period-Cohort Analysis," *American Sociological Review* 73, no. 2 (April 2008): 204–26.

5. https://www.psychologytoday.com/us/blog/changepower/201501/older-happier-5-amazing-findings-recent-research.

7. DISCOVERING OUR PARENTS MAY NEED TO LEAVE HOME

1. This was phased out under the Affordable Care Act.

2. The Centers for Disease Control defines aging in place as "the ability to live in one's own home and community safely, independently, and comfortably, regardless of age, income, or ability level." For additional information, see chapter 8.

8. FINDING THE BEST FIT FOR OUR PARENTS' NEW HOME

1. From the 1924 Buddy DeSylva and Joseph Meyer song, written for the 1921 Broadway musical *Bombo*, starring Al Jolson and published by Brunswick Music.

2. See, for example, the *Time* magazine, January 17, 2005, special issue, "The Science of Happiness."

3. To check if your parents qualify for this program, no matter if they are living in their own homes or in an assisted-living facility, go to https://www.veteranaid.org.

4. Check online at http://www.Pace4you.org for those conditions and the benefits available.

5. Although this term also represents a philosophical position about people with disabilities, when we're speaking in this eldercare context, IL is a step on the continuum of care requirements with assisted living—help from others—being the next rung up of care.

9. DEALING WITH ALL OUR PARENTS' STUFF

1. Jack revealed some of his patriotic ideals in his songs. One of these, coauthored with Robert Colby, was called "The American Dream," and it was the theme song for a major New York Festival starring Howard Keel.

10. SETTLING OUR PARENTS INTO THEIR NEW LIVES

1. From "New York, New York," written by John Kander and Fred Ebb and published by EMI/Uniart Catalog, Inc.

11. TRYING TO MAKE A PERMANENT POPLAN

1. See "Falls and the Elderly," Netwellness, http://www.netwellness.org/healthtopics/aging/faq9.cfm.

2. J. A. Stevens, "Fatalities and Injuries from Falls among Older Adults—United States, 1993–2003 and 2001–2005," *Morbidity and Mortality Weekly Report* 55, no. 45 (2006): 1221–24.

3. I. P. Donald and C. J. Bulpitt, "The Prognosis of Falls in Elderly People Living at Home," *Age and Ageing* 28 (1999): 121–25.

4. B. J. Vellas, S. J. Wayne, L. J. Romero, R. N. Baumgartner, and P. J. Garry, "Fear of Falling and Restriction of Mobility in Elderly Fallers," *Age and Aging* 26 (1997): 189–93.

13. TURNING POP INTO OUR GIANT DO-OVER

1. These are programs aiming to help people recover from their addictive and compulsive behaviors. Based upon spiritual principles, the programs involve a series of steps, including making an inventory of troubling past behaviors and seeking amends. They were originally proposed by Bill W and Alcoholics Anonymous (AA).

2. A new survey from the National Family Caregivers Association shows a much more even split than the historical numbers of 75 percent or more who were women. Today: 56 percent female, 44 percent male. Fifty-two percent of the survey's respondents, 39 percent of whom were men, stated they provided physical care, including help with dressing, bathing, toileting, eating, and mobility. Forty-six percent of respondents, 41 percent of them men, reported being involved in performing nursing activity such as managing medications, changing dressings, or monitoring vital signs. CelebrateLove.com, "November: National Family Caregivers Month," http://www.celebratelove.com/caregivers.htm.

15. DOING THE ONLY THING LEFT

1. Barack Obama, *Dreams of My Father* (New York: Crown, 2007).

2. For more information about Jack Wolf's music, go to http://mpcamusicpublishing.com/catalog/artists-songwriters/jack-wolf-integrity-music.

3. You will want to check that regulations and offerings have not changed in the interim, since this book's publication. You can contact Medicare directly or go online to: www.medicare.gov/Publications/Pubs/pdf/11386.pdf.

16. LETTING GO OF THE BELOVED PARENTS WE'VE PARENTED

1. Ernest Holmes, *The Science of Mind* (New York: G. P. Putnam's Sons, 1926).

2. http://www.scienceofminduk.org/believe_faq.html#15.

3. Judy Collins, "In the Twilight," on *Bohemian* (New York: Wildflower Records, 2011).

4. By the time I was writing this chapter, Sue had unfortunately also died. She was two months younger than me. Though she is gone, she still "tells" me not to waste time while I am still on the planet.

5. William Wordsworth, "Splendour in the Grass."

17. WHEN POP IS OVER AND WE NEED TO LAUNCH OUR NEW LIVES

1. From the song, "Me and Bobby McGee," written by Kris Kristofferson and Fred Foster, published by EMI Music.

2. Tom Robbins, *Still Life with Woodpecker* (New York: Bantam, 1980).

ACKNOWLEDGMENTS

I have learned that nothing of any real importance is created alone: there are always many people who contribute. That adage is well borne out in your having this book to read.

Key people worked diligently, lovingly, and wisely in developing this to become a published work of bibliotherapy—therapeutic learning from reading—and thereby available to guide seventy-five million families through their POPcycles. I am so grateful to them:

Murray Weiss, my wonderful literary agent, at Catalyst Literary Management, who tirelessly insisted that this book be published and, because of him, we found Rowman & Littlefield.

Rowman & Littlefield, my encouraging and enthusiastic publisher and Suzanne I. Staszak-Silva, my editor there, and other staff there who saw the value in this book and had a vision that they carefully pursued throughout the process. Those involved in the editing, graphics, publishing, and printing teams.

Bridget Doshi, whose service as part of our POPteam has been loyal and deeply valued.

My original family, Jack and Lillian Geist Wolf, who gave unceasingly of their heartfelt gifts: the generosity of their time, attention, and resources. All they did and said, as well as what they did not do or say, all got me to here. I am so grateful! My folks consistently expressed pride in my accomplishments and encouraged making my own choices, even if they'd have done things differently. And, during their later years, when they were increasingly vulnerable, they confirmed their ultimate confidence in me by allowing me to POParent them. I hope they knew how much that meant to me.

I have been privileged to learn and be part of several families—in addition to the Wolfs and the Geists. The Eldridge clan, the Waterman crew, and the Frances families have each been major influences on me and my understanding of families.

To those many teachers who arrived in my life when I needed them most, wearing their various "hats," I am so grateful to you:

My dear patients, extraordinary and long-standing friends, and caring colleagues who invited me to listen to their POP stories, listened to mine, encouraged me to write this book and get it published, when I was still hesitant.

Dr. Rick Moss, my adopted brother, his parents, my Aunt Miriam, and many others from my families.

Dr. Ernest Holmes and his spiritual teachings; Reverends Michael Beckwith and Terry Cole-Whittaker and Ram Dass.

Werner Erhard; the scholars I call "happiness scientists"; the "attachment theory" people; and my mentor, office partner, and dear friend, the late Dr. Michael McGrail.

The people who helped me POParent Lillian and Jack, all part of our TEAM POP: lawyers, accountants, dentists, audiologists, doctors, devoted caregivers, caring staffs at numerous facilities, and most especially the patient and kind Florence Walkes.

Most of all, I wish to thank and fully acknowledge my beloved partner, husband, and finest friend, Andrew Frances. As my manager and editor, he helped me stay focused on the big picture, tirelessly edited this book, promoted the manuscript, helped create the POP website, and found me Murray Weiss. His loving consistency, thoroughness, energy, and vision have been irreplaceable in bringing this book to you; and his love, generosity, and kindness have expanded my understanding of how journeying through life with loving family truly transforms us all.

SUGGESTED READING

Chopra, Deepak. *Ageless Body, Timeless Mind: The Quantum Alternative to Growing Old*. New York: Crown, 1993.

Gawande, Atul. *Being Mortal: Medicine and What Matters in the End*. New York: Henry Holt, 2014.

Gibbons, Leeza. *Take Your Oxygen First: Protecting Your Health and Happiness While Caring for a Loved One with Memory Loss*. Brooklyn, NY: LaChance, 2009.

Hoffman, Sharona. *Aging with a Plan: How a Little Thought Today Can Vastly Improve Your Tomorrow*. Santa Barbara, CA: Praeger, 2015.

Irving, Paul H. *The Upside of Aging: How Long Life Is Changing the World of Health, Work, Innovation, Policy, and Purpose*. Hoboken, NJ: John Wiley and Sons, 2014.

Kübler-Ross, Elisabeth, and David Kessler. *On Grief and Grieving: Finding the Meaning of Grief through the Five Stages of Loss*. New York: Scribner, 2005.

Lipton, Bruce H. *The Biology of Belief: Unleashing the Power of Consciousness, Matter and Miracles*. n.p.: Authors Publishing Corp., 2005.

Northrup, Christiane. *Goddesses Never Age: The Secret Prescription for Radiance, Vitality, and Well-Being*. Carlsbad, CA: Hay House, 2015.

Schachter-Shalomi, Zalman, and Ronald S. Miller. *From Age-ing to Sage-ing: A Revolutionary Approach to Growing Older*. New York: Warner Books, 1995.

Weil, Andrew. *Healthy Aging: A Lifelong Guide to Your Well-Being*. New York: Knopf, 2005.

INDEX

ABOUT THE AUTHOR

Jane Wolf Frances, MSW, JD, Master POP (ParentingOurParents) Family Coach, has counseled thousands of families to successfully resolve their life cycle challenges—emotional, legal, and practical. Now, she shares her own solo journey and the solutions she found, both personal and in building community. In addition to writing this book, she has published articles in the *California Bar Journal*, in legal and drug abuse professional periodicals, and a chapter in a book on what constitutes "success." She also has a well-read blog for more than five years at www.ParentingOurParents.org.